Introductory Adaptive Trial Designs

A Practical Guide with R

Chapman & Hall/CRC Biostatistics Series

Editor-in-Chief

Shein-Chung Chow, Ph.D., Professor, Department of Biostatistics and Bioinformatics,
Duke University School of Medicine, Durham, North Carolina

Series Editors

Byron Jones, Biometrical Fellow, Statistical Methodology, Integrated Information Sciences,
Novartis Pharma AG, Basel, Switzerland

Jen-pei Liu, Professor, Division of Biometry, Department of Agronomy,
National Taiwan University, Taipei, Taiwan

Karl E. Peace, Georgia Cancer Coalition, Distinguished Cancer Scholar, Senior Research Scientist
and Professor of Biostatistics, Jiann-Ping Hsu College of Public Health,
Georgia Southern University, Statesboro, Georgia

Bruce W. Turnbull, Professor, School of Operations Research and Industrial Engineering,
Cornell University, Ithaca, New York

Published Titles

Adaptive Design Methods in Clinical Trials, Second Edition
Shein-Chung Chow and Mark Chang

Adaptive Designs for Sequential Treatment Allocation
Alessandro Baldi Antognini and Alessandra Giovagnoli

Adaptive Design Theory and Implementation Using SAS and R, Second Edition
Mark Chang

Advanced Bayesian Methods for Medical Test Accuracy
Lyle D. Broemeling

Advances in Clinical Trial Biostatistics
Nancy L. Geller

Applied Meta-Analysis with R
Ding-Geng (Din) Chen and Karl E. Peace

Basic Statistics and Pharmaceutical Statistical Applications, Second Edition
James E. De Muth

Bayesian Adaptive Methods for Clinical Trials
Scott M. Berry, Bradley P. Carlin, J. Jack Lee, and Peter Muller

Bayesian Analysis Made Simple: An Excel GUI for WinBUGS
Phil Woodward

Bayesian Methods for Measures of Agreement
Lyle D. Broemeling

Bayesian Methods in Epidemiology
Lyle D. Broemeling

Bayesian Methods in Health Economics
Gianluca Baio

Bayesian Missing Data Problems: EM, Data Augmentation and Noniterative Computation
Ming T. Tan, Guo-Liang Tian, and Kai Wang Ng

Bayesian Modeling in Bioinformatics
Dipak K. Dey, Samiran Ghosh, and Bani K. Mallick

Benefit-Risk Assessment in Pharmaceutical Research and Development
Andreas Sashegyi, James Felli, and Rebecca Noel

Biosimilars: Design and Analysis of Follow-on Biologics
Shein-Chung Chow

Biostatistics: A Computing Approach
Stewart J. Anderson

Causal Analysis in Biomedicine and Epidemiology: Based on Minimal Sufficient Causation
Mikel Aickin

Clinical and Statistical Considerations in Personalized Medicine
Claudio Carini, Sandeep Menon, and Mark Chang

Chapman & Hall/CRC Biostatistics Series

Introductory Adaptive Trial Designs

A Practical Guide with R

Mark Chang

AMAG Pharmaceuticals, Inc
Lexington, Massachusetts, USA

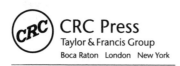

CRC Press
Taylor & Francis Group
Boca Raton   London   New York

CRC Press is an imprint of the
Taylor & Francis Group, an **informa** business

A CHAPMAN & HALL BOOK

CRC Press
Taylor & Francis Group
6000 Broken Sound Parkway NW, Suite 300
Boca Raton, FL 33487-2742

© 2015 by Taylor & Francis Group, LLC
CRC Press is an imprint of Taylor & Francis Group, an Informa business

No claim to original U.S. Government works

Printed on acid-free paper
Version Date: 20150505

International Standard Book Number-13: 978-1-4987-1746-5 (Hardback)

Visit the Taylor & Francis Web site at
http://www.taylorandfrancis.com

and the CRC Press Web site at
http://www.crcpress.com

Contents

Preface

The second version of my book, *Adaptive Design Theory and Implementation Using SAS and R*, was just expanded from 350 pages to nearly 700 pages; however, it still cannot catch up with the development of research of adaptive clinical trials. On the other hand, with the popular increase of adaptive trials, there has been an increase in demand for a tutorial book, which can help newcomers quickly get a feel of adaptive designs and grasp the foundations of adaptive design methods without having to commit a huge amount of time and effort. This *Introductory Adaptive Trial Designs with R* was written for this purpose. We made this a tutorial style book, reducing the mathematics to a minimum, and making it as practical as possible. Instead of providing the black-box-like general commercial software packages, I have developed the R functions and included them in the book for readers to better understand the algorithms and to be able to customize the adaptive designs to meet their needs. By learning through doing, the reader doesn't need to buy any software package, but instead can download the popular freeware R and do adaptive design immediately. For those who do not have any experience with R, we have provided a 30 minute tutorial in Appendix A.

To learn adaptive designs effectively, the reader should run the simulations for all the examples provided in the book and change the input parameters to see how each input parameter will affect the simulation outcomes or design operating characteristics.

I hope you have a very enjoyable experience learning adaptive trial designs; the knowledge you acquire can be used in your work and your research immediately.

Mark Chang

Chapter 1

Introduction

1.1 Motivation

The rapidly escalating costs and increasing failure rate in drug development decrease willingness and ability to bring many candidates forward into the clinic. There are multiple reasons: (1) Those "low-hanging fruit" in the chemical compound space have already been picked, (2) due to ethical considerations, a pivotal clinical trial cannot be a placebo-controlled trial when a drug for the disease is available; however, an active-controlled, in which the test drug is compared against the best drug in the market, makes the efficacy margin much smaller than in a placebo-controlled trial. However, the regulatory agencies in general still require type-I error rates of at most 5%, although the meaning of the type-I error is completely different: one is compared to placebo and the other is compared to active drug. Thus a diminished margin for improvement escalates the level of difficulty in statistically proving drug benefits or the sample size must increase, as must the cost and time. To stay in competition, many pharmaceutical companies adopt different strategies, such as company mergers or acquisitions, late phase outsourcing, reducing workforce in the early research but buying promising compounds that are ready for clinical trials. In addition to implementations of strategies in business, there is also a significant change in the technological side: a paradigm shift from classical statistic clinical trial designs to adaptive designs, which can lead to a reduction in cost and time, and an increase in success rate in drug development. In this chapter, we will review commonly used adaptive designs and questions and answers that a newcomer may have.

1.2 Adaptive Designs in Clinical Trials

An adaptive design is a clinical trial design that allows adaptations or modifications to aspects of the trial after its initiation without undermining the validity and integrity of the trial (Chow, Chang, and Pong, 2005). The PhRMA

1

Working Group defines an adaptive design as a clinical study design that uses accumulating data to decide how to modify aspects of the study as it continues, without undermining the validity and integrity of the trial (Gallo et al., 2006; Dragalin and Fedorov 2006).

The adaptive designs may include, but are not limited to (1) a group sequential design, (2) a sample-size reestimation design, (3) a drop-arm design, (4) an add-arm design, (5) a biomarker-adaptive design, (6) an adaptive randomization design, and (7) an adaptive dose-escalation design. An adaptive design usually consists of multiple stages. At each stage, data analyses are conducted, and adaptations are mode based on updated information to maximize the probability of success.

1.2.1   *Group Sequential Design*

A group sequential design (GSD) is an adaptive design that allows a trial due to stop earlier based on the results of interim analyses. For a trial with a positive result, early stopping ensures that a new drug product can be available to the patients sooner. If a negative result is indicated, early stopping avoids wasting resources and reduces the unnecessary exposure to the ineffective drug. Sequential methods typically lead to savings in sample-size, time, and cost when compared with the classical design with a fixed sample-size. GSD is probably one of the most commonly used adaptive designs in clinical trials.

There are three different types of GSDs: early efficacy stopping design, early futility stopping design, and early efficacy or futility stopping design. If we believe (based on prior knowledge) that the test treatment is very promising, then an early efficacy stopping design should be used. If we are very concerned that the test treatment may not work, an early futility stopping design should be employed. If we are not certain about the magnitude of the effect size, a GSD permitting early stopping for both efficacy and futility should be considered.

1.2.2   *Sample-Size Reestimation Design*

A sample-size reestimation (SSR) design refers to an adaptive design that allows for sample-size adjustment or reestimation based on the review of interim analysis results (Figure 1.1). The sample-size requirement for a trial is sensitive to the treatment effect and its variability. An inaccurate estimation of the effect size and its variability could lead to an underpowered or overpowered design, neither of which is desirable. If a trial is underpowered, it will be unlikely to detect a clinically meaningful difference, and consequently could prevent a potentially effective drug from being delivered to patients. On the other hand, if a trial is overpowered, it could lead to unnecessary exposure

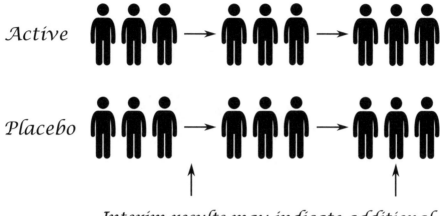

Active

Placebo

Interim results may indicate additional patients required to preserve the power

Figure 1.1: Sample-Size Reestimation Design

of many patients to a potentially harmful compound when the drug, in fact, is not practically effective. In practice, it is often difficult to estimate the effect size and variability when we design a clinical trial protocol. Thus, it is desirable to have the flexibility to reestimate the sample-size in the middle of the trial.

There are three types of sample-size reestimation procedures, namely, SSR based on blinded data, SSR based on unblinded data, and the mixed approach. If the sample size adjustment is based on the (observed) pooled variance at the interim analysis to recalculate the required sample-size, it does not require unblinding the data. If the effect size and its variability are re-assessed, and sample-size is adjusted based on the updated information. The mixed approach also requires unblinded data, but does not fully use the unblinded information, thus providing an information masker to the public (see Chapter 5). The statistical method for adjustment could be based on effect size or the conditional power.

A GSD can also be viewed as a SSR design, in which the sample size increase is predetermined. For example if pass the interim analysis, the sample size will to the second stage sample size regardless of effect size. However, when the SSR trial passes the interim analysis, the sample size is usually determined by the observed effect size at interim and the so-called conditional power.

1.2.3 Drop-Arm Design

A drop-arm or drop-loser design (DLD) is an adaptive design consisting of multiple stages. At each stage, interim analyses are performed and the losers

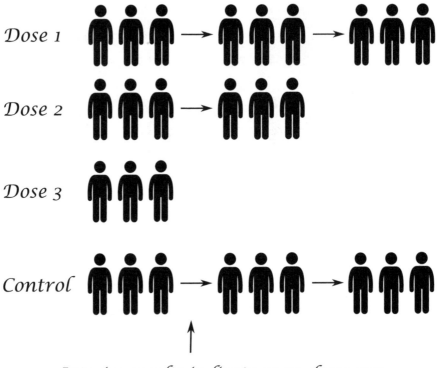

Dose 1

Dose 2

Dose 3

Control

Interim results indicate some doses are inferior and can be dropped from the study

Figure 1.2:   Drop-Arm Design

(i.e., inferior treatment groups) are dropped based on prespecified criteria (Figure 1.2). Ultimately, the best arm(s) are retained. If there is a control group, it is usually retained for the purpose of comparison. This type of design can be used in phase-II/III combined trials. A phase-II clinical trial is often a dose-response study, where the goal is to assess whether there is a treatment effect. If there is a treatment effect, the goal becomes finding the appropriate dose level (or treatment groups) for the phase-III trials. This type of traditional design is not efficient with respect to time and resources because the phase-II efficacy data are not pooled with data from phase-III trials, which are the pivotal trials for confirming efficacy. Therefore, it is desirable to combine phases II and III so that the data can be used efficiently, and the time required for drug development can be reduced.

1.2.4 *Add-Arm Design*

In a classical drop-loser design, patients are randomized into all arms (doses) and, at the interim analysis, inferior arms are dropped. Therefore, compared to the traditional dose-finding design, this adaptive design can reduce the sample size by not carrying over all doses to the end of the trial or dropping the losers earlier. However, all the doses have to be explored. For unimodal (including linear or umbrella) response curves, we proposed an effective dose-finding design that allows adding arms at the interim analysis. The trial design starts with two arms; depending on the response of the two arms and the unimodality assumption, we can decide which new arms to add. This design does not require exploring all arms (doses) to find the best responsive dose; therefore it can further reduce the sample size from the drop-loser design by as much as 10%–20% (Chang and Wang, 2014)

1.2.5 *Adaptive Randomization Design*

An adaptive randomization design (ARD) allows modification of randomization schedules during the conduct of the trial. In clinical trials, randomization is commonly used to ensure a balance with respect to patient characteristics among treatment groups. However, there is another type of ARD, called response-adaptive randomization (RAR), in which the allocation probability is based on the response of the previous patients. RAR was initially proposed because of ethical considerations (i.e., to have a larger probability to allocate patients to a superior treatment group); however, response randomization can be considered a drop-loser design with a seamless allocation probability of shifting from an inferior arm to a superior arm. The well-known response-adaptive models include the randomized play-the-winner (RPW) model.

1.2.6 *Biomarker-Enrichment Design*

Biomarker-adaptive design (BAD) or biomarker-enrichment design (BED) refers to a design that allows for adaptations using information obtained from biomarkers. A biomarker is a characteristic that is objectively measured and evaluated as an indicator of normal biologic or pathogenic processes or pharmacological response to a therapeutic intervention (Chakravarty, 2005). A biomarker can be a classifier, prognostic, or predictive marker.

A classifier biomarker is a marker that usually does not change over the course of the study, like DNA markers. Classifier biomarkers can be used to select the most appropriate target population, or even for personalized treatment. Classifier markers can also be used in other situations. For example, it is often the case that a pharmaceutical company has to make a decision

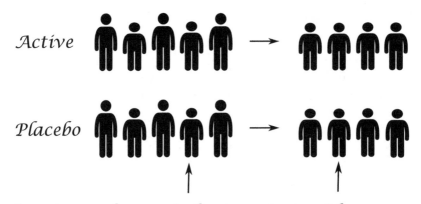

Active

Placebo

Interim results may indicate patients with gene x are much more responsive to the drug; therefore at the second stage only patients with gene x will be recruited.

Figure 1.3:   Biomarker-Adaptive Design

whether to target a very selective population for whom the test drug likely works well or to target a broader population for whom the test drug is less likely to work well. However, the size of the selective population may be too small to justify the overall benefit to the patient population. In this case, a BAD may be used, where the biomarker response at interim analysis can be used to determine which target populations should be focused on (Figure 1.3).

1.2.7   *Adaptive Dose-Escalation Design*

Dose-escalation is often considered in early phases of clinical development for identifying maximum tolerated dose (MTD), which is often considered the optimal dose for later phases of clinical development. An adaptive dose-escalation design is a design at which the dose level used to treat the next-entered patient is dependent on the toxicity of the previous patients, based on some traditional escalation rules. Many early dose-escalation rules such as 3+3 rules are adaptive, but the adaptation algorithm is somewhat ad hoc. Recently more advanced dose-escalation rules have been developed using modeling approaches (frequentist or Bayesian framework) such as the continual reassessment method (CRM) (O'Quigley et al., 1990; Chang and Chow, 2005) and other accelerated escalation algorithms. These algorithms can reduce the sample-size and overall toxicity in a trial and improve the accuracy and precision of the estimation of the MTD.

1.3 Clinical Trial Simulation

CTS was started in the early 1970s and became popular in the mid-1990s due to increased computing power. Clinical trial simulation (CTS) is a process that mimics clinical trials using computer programs. CTS is particularly important in adaptive designs for several reasons: (1) the statistical theory of adaptive design is complicated with limited analytical solutions available under certain assumptions; (2) the concept of CTS is very intuitive and easy to implement; (3) CTS can be used to model very complicated situations with minimum assumptions, and type-I errors can be strongly controlled; (4) using CTS, we not only can calculate the power of an adaptive design, but can also generate many other important operating characteristics such as expected sample-size, conditional power, and repeated confidence interval; ultimately this leads to the selection of an optimal trial design or clinical development plan; (5) CTS can be used to study the validity and robustness of an adaptive design in different hypothetical clinical settings, or with protocol deviations; (6) CTS can be used to monitor trials, project outcomes, anticipate problems, and suggest remedies before it is too late; (7) CTS can be used to visualize the dynamic trial process from patient recruitment, drug distribution, treatment administration, and pharmacokinetic processes to biomarkers and clinical responses; and, finally, (8) CTS has minimal cost associated with it and can be done in a short time.

1.4 Characteristics of Adaptive Designs

Adaptive design is a sequential data-driven approach. It is a dynamic process that allows for real-time learning. It is flexible and allows for modifications to the trial, which make the design cost-efficient and robust against the failure. Adaptive design is a systematic way to design different phases of trials, thus streamlining and optimizing the drug development process. In contrast, the traditional approach is composed of weakly connected phasewise processes. Adaptive design is a decision-oriented, sequential learning process that requires up-front planning and a great deal of collaboration among the different parties involved in the drug development process. To this end, Bayesian methodology and computer simulation play important roles. Finally, the flexibility of adaptive design does not compromise the validity and integrity of the trial or the development process.

There are many different adaptive designs we can choose. What is the overall process of an adaptive design approach? Figure 1.4 gives a overview of the adaptive trial flow chart. Further details can be found in Chapter 12.

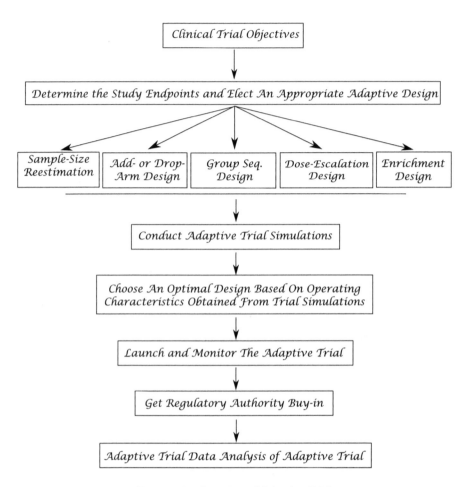

Figure 1.4:   Overview of Adaptive Trial

Adaptive design methods represent a revolution in pharmaceutical research and development. Using adaptive designs, we can increase the chances for success of a trial with a reduced cost. Bayesian approaches provide an ideal tool for optimizing trial designs and development plans. Clinical trial simulations offer a powerful tool to design and monitor trials. Adaptive design, the Bayesian approach, and trial simulation combine to form an ultimate statistical instrument for the most successful drug development programs.

1.5   FAQs about Adaptive Designs

In recent years, scientific journalists and colleagues from the industry and academia asked some questions about adaptive designs. I present a few of them in the following:

1. *What challenges does the adaptive trial model present?*

First, statistical methods are available for most common adaptive designs, but for more complicated adaptive designs, the methodologies are still in development.

Operationally, an adaptive design often requires real-time or near real-time data collection and analysis. In this regard, data standardizations, such as CDISC and electronic data capture (EDC), are very helpful in data cleaning and reconciliation. Note that not all adaptive designs require perfectly clean data at interim analysis, but the cleaner the data are, the more efficient the design is. Adaptive designs require the ability to rapidly integrate knowledge and experiences from different disciplines into the decision-making process and hence require a shift to a more collaborative working environment among disciplines.

From a regulatory standpoint, there is no regulatory guidance for adaptive designs at the moment, but the draft of the guidance of adaptive design was released in 2010. Therefore, at the moment, adaptive trials are reviewed on a case-by-case basis. Naturally there are fears that a protocol using this innovative approach may be rejected, causing a delay.

Regulatory documents related to the adaptive clinical trials were issued during 2007 to 2012. They are:

(1) European Medicines Agency (EMA) – Reflection Paper on Methodological Issues in Confirmatory Clinical Trials Planned with an Adaptive Design (October 2007)

(2) US Food and Drug Administration (FDA) – Draft Guidance – Guidance for Industry Adaptive Design Clinical Trials for Drugs and Biologics (February 2010)

(3) US Food and Drug Administration (FDA) – Guidance for the Use of Bayesian Statistics in Medical Device Clinical Trials (February 2010)

(4) US Food and Drug Administration (FDA) – Draft Guidance – Guidance for Industry on Enrichment Strategies for Clinical Trials to Support Approval of Human Drugs and Biological Products (December 2012)

The interim unblinding may potentially cause bias and put the integrity of the trial at risk. Therefore, the unblinding procedure should be well established before the trial starts, and frequent unblinding should be avoided. Also, unblinding the premature results to the public could jeopardize the trial.

2. *How would adaptive trials affect traditional phases of drug development? How are safety and efficacy measured in this type of trial?*

Adaptive designs change the way we conduct clinical trials. Trials in different phases can be combined to create a seamless study. The final safety and efficacy requirements are not reduced because of adaptive designs. In fact, with adaptive designs, the efficacy and safety signals are collected and reviewed earlier and more often than in traditional designs. Therefore, we may have a better chance of avoiding unsafe drug exposure to large patient populations. A phase-II and -III combined seamless design, when the trial is carried out to the final stage, has longer term patient efficacy and safety data than traditional phase-II and phase-III trials; however, precautions should be taken at the interim decision-making when data are not mature.

3. *What are some differences between adaptive trials and the traditional trial model with respect to the supply of clinical trial materials?*

For a traditional or classical design, the amount of material required is fixed and can be easily planned before the trial starts. However, for some adaptive trials, the exact amount of required materials is not clear until later stages of the trial. Also, the next dosage for a site may not be fully determined until the time of randomization; therefore, vendors may need to develop a better drug distribution strategy.

4. *What areas of clinical development would experience cost/time savings with the adaptive trial model?*

Adaptive design can be used in any phase, even in the preclinical and discovery phases. Drug discovery and development is a sequence of decision processes. The traditional paradigm breaks this into weakly connected fragments or phases. An adaptive approach will eventually be utilized for the whole development process to get the right drug to the right patient at the right time.

Adaptive design may require fewer patients, less trial material, sometimes fewer lab tests, less work for data collection, and fewer data queries to be resolved. However, an adaptive trial requires much more time during up-front planning and simulation studies.

Chapter 2

Classical Design

2.1 Introduction

Pharmaceutical medicine uses all the scientific, clinical, statistical, regulatory, and business knowledge available to provide a challenging and rewarding career. On average, it costs about $1.8 billion to take a new compound to market and only one in 10,000 compounds ever reaches the market. There are three major phases of drug development: (1) preclinical research and development, (2) clinical research and development, and (3) after the compound is on the market, a possible "post-marketing" phase.

Clinical trials are usually divided into three phases. The primary objectives of phase I are to (1) determine the metabolism and pharmacological activities of the drug, the side effects associated with increasing dose, and early evidence of effectiveness, and (2) to obtain sufficient information regarding the drug's pharmacokinetics and pharmacological effects to permit the design of well-controlled and scientifically valid phase-II clinical studies (21 CFR 312.21). Unless it is an oncology study, where the maximum tolerated dose (MTD) is primarily determined by a phase-I dose-escalation study, the dose-response or dose-finding study is usually conducted in phase II, and efficacy is usually the main focus. The choice of study design and study population in a dose-response trial will depend on the phase of development, therapeutic indication under investigation, and severity of the disease in the patient population of interest (ICH Guideline E4, 1994). Phase-III trials are considered confirmatory trials.

The FDA does not actually approve the drug itself for sale. It approves the labeling and the package insert. United States law requires truth in labeling, and the FDA ensures that claims that a drug is safe and effective for treatment of a specified disease or condition have, in fact, been proven. All prescription drugs must have labels, and without proof of the truth of its label, a drug may not be sold in the United States.

In classical trial designs, power and sample-size calculations are a major task. The sample-size calculations for two-group designs have been studied by many scholars, among them Julious (2004), Chow et al.(2003), Machin et al. (1997), Campbell et al. (1995), and Lachin and Foukes (1986).

In what follows, we will review a unified formulation for sample-size calculation in classical two-arm designs including superiority, noninferiority, and equivalence trials.

2.2   Two-Group Superiority

When testing a null hypothesis $H_0 : \varepsilon \leq 0$ against an alternative hypothesis $H_a : \varepsilon > 0$, where ε is the treatment effect (difference in response), the type-I error rate function is defined as

$$\alpha = \Pr \left\{ \text{reject } H_0 \text{ when } H_0 \text{ is true} \right\}.$$

Similarly, the type-II error rate function β is defined as

$$\beta = \Pr \left\{ \text{fail to reject } H_0 \text{ when } H_a \text{ is true} \right\}.$$

For example, for the null hypothesis $H_0 : \mu_2 - \mu_1 \leq 0$, where μ_1 and μ_2 are the means of the two treatment groups, the maximum type-I error rate occurs on the boundary of H_0 when $\mu_2 - \mu_1 = 0$. Let $T = \frac{\hat{\mu}_2 - \hat{\mu}_1}{\hat{\sigma}}$, where $\hat{\mu}_i$ and $\hat{\sigma}$ are the sample mean and pooled sample standard deviation, respectively. Further, let $\Phi_o(T)$ denote the cumulative distribution function (c.d.f.) of the test statistic on the boundary of the null hypothesis domain, i.e., when $\varepsilon = 0$, and let $\Phi_a(T)$ denote the c.d.f. under H_a. Given this information, under the large sample assumption, $\Phi_o(T)$ is the c.d.f. of the standard normal distribution, $N(0, 1)$, and $\Phi_a(T)$ is the c.d.f. of $N(\frac{\sqrt{n}\varepsilon}{2\sigma}, 1)$, where n is the total sample-size and σ is the common standard deviation (Figure 2.1).

The power of the test statistic T under a particular H_a can be expressed as follows:

$$\text{Power}(\varepsilon) = \Pr(T \geq z_{1-\alpha} | H_a),$$

which is equivalent to

$$\text{Power}(\varepsilon) = \Phi \left(\frac{\sqrt{n}\varepsilon}{2\sigma} - z_{1-\alpha} \right), \tag{2.1}$$

where Φ is the c.d.f. of the standard normal distribution, ε is treatment difference, and $z_{1-\beta}$ and $z_{1-\alpha}$ are the percentiles of the standard normal distribution. The total sample-size is given by

$$n = \frac{4(z_{1-\alpha} + z_{1-\beta})^2 \sigma^2}{\varepsilon^2}. \tag{2.2}$$

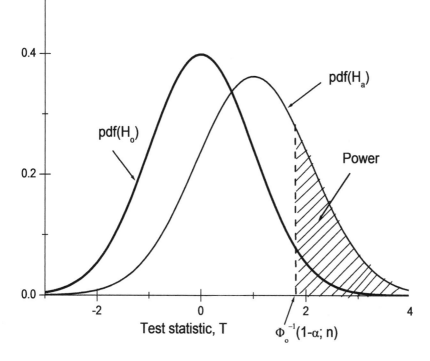

Figure 2.1: Power as a Function of α and n

More generally, for an imbalanced design with sample-size ratio $r = n_1/n_2$ and a margin δ ($\delta > 0$ for superiority test and $\delta < 0$ for noninferiority test), the sample-size is given by

$$n_2 = \frac{(z_{1-\alpha} + z_{1-\beta})^2 \sigma^2 (1 + 1/r)}{(\varepsilon - \delta)^2}. \tag{2.3}$$

Equation (2.3) is a general sample-size formulation for the two-group designs with a normal, binary, or survival endpoint. When using the formulation, the corresponding "standard deviation" σ should be used, examples of which have been listed in Table 2.1 for commonly used endpoints (Chang and Chow, 2006).

Example 2.1 Arteriosclerotic Vascular Disease Trial

Cholesterol is the main lipid associated with arteriosclerotic vascular disease. The purpose of cholesterol testing is to identify patients at risk for arteriosclerotic heart disease. The liver metabolizes cholesterol to its free form and transports it to the bloodstream via lipoproteins. Nearly 75% of the cholesterol is bound to low-density lipoproteins (LDLs) – "bad cholesterol" – and 25% is bound to high-density lipoproteins (HDLs) – "good cholesterol." Therefore, cholesterol is the main component of LDLs and only a minimal

Table 2.1: Sample Sizes for Different Types of Endpoints

Endpoint	Sample-Size	Variance
One mean	$n = \frac{(z_{1-a}+z_{1-\beta})^2 \sigma^2}{\varepsilon^2}$;	
Two means	$n_1 = \frac{(z_{1-a}+z_{1-\beta})^2 \sigma^2}{(1+1/r)^{-1}\varepsilon^2}$;	
One proportion	$n = \frac{(z_{1-a}+z_{1-\beta})^2 \sigma^2}{\varepsilon^2}$;	$\sigma^2 = p(1-p)$
Two proportions	$n_1 = \frac{(z_{1-a}+z_{1-\beta})^2 \sigma^2}{(1+1/r)^{-1}\varepsilon^2}$;	$\sigma^2 = \bar{p}(1-\bar{p})$; $\bar{p} = \frac{n_1 p_1 + n_2 p_2}{n_1 + n_2}$.
One survival curve	$n = \frac{(z_{1-a}+z_{1-\beta})^2 \sigma^2}{\varepsilon^2}$;	$\sigma^2 = \lambda_0^2 \left(1 - \frac{e^{\lambda_0 T_0}-1}{T_0 \lambda_0 e^{\lambda_0 T_s}}\right)^{-1}$
Two survival curves	$n_1 = \frac{(z_{1-a}+z_{1-\beta})^2 \sigma^2}{(1+1/r)^{-1}\varepsilon^2}$;	$\sigma^2 = \frac{r\sigma_1^2+\sigma_2^2}{1+r}$, $\sigma_i^2 = \lambda_i^2 \left(1 - \frac{e^{\lambda_i T_0}-1}{T_0 \lambda_i e^{\lambda_i T_s}}\right)^{-1}$

Note: $r = \frac{n_2}{n_1}$. $\lambda_0 =$ expected hazard rate, $T_0 =$ uniform patient accrual time and $T_s =$ trial duration. Logrank-test is used for comparison of the two survival curves.

component of HDLs. LDL is the substance most directly associated with increased risk of coronary heart disease (CHD).

Suppose we are interested in a trial for evaluating the effect of a test drug on cholesterol in patients with CHD. A two-group parallel design is chosen for the trial with LDL as the primary endpoint. The treatment difference in LDL is estimated to be 5% with a standard deviation of 0.3. For power = 90% and one-sided $\alpha = 0.025$, the total sample can be calculated using (2.2):

$$n = \frac{4(1.96 + 1.28)^2 \left(0.3^2\right)}{0.05^2} = 1512.$$

2.3 Two-Group Noninferiority Trial

As the European regulatory agency, Committee for Medicinal Products for Human Use (CHMP, 2005), stated, "Many clinical trials comparing a test product with an active comparator are designed as noninferiority trials. The term 'noninferiority' is now well established, but if taken literally could be misleading. The objective of a noninferiority trial is sometimes stated as being to demonstrate that the test product is not inferior to the comparator. However, only a superiority trial can demonstrate this. In fact a noninferiority trial aims to demonstrate that the test product is not worse than the comparator by more than a pre-specified, small amount. This amount is known as the noninferiority margin, or delta."

Until recent years, the majority of clinical trials were designed for superiority to a comparative drug (the control group). A statistic shows that only 23% of all NDAs from 1998 to 2002 were innovative drugs, and the rest were accounted for as "me-too" drugs (Chang, 2010). The "me-too" drugs are judged based on noninferiority criteria. The increasing popularity of noninferiority trials is a reflection of regulatory and industry adjustments in response to increasing challenges in drug development.

There are three major sources of uncertainty about the conclusions from a noninferiority (NI) study: (1) the uncertainty of the active-control effect over a placebo, which is estimated from historical data; (2) the possibility that the control effect may change over time, violating the "constancy assumption"; and (3) the risk of making a wrong decision from the test of the noninferiority hypothesis in the NI study, i.e., the type-I error. These three uncertainties have to be considered in developing a noninferiority design method.

Most commonly used noninferiority trials are based on parallel, two-group designs with fixed noninferiority margins:

$$H_0 : \mu_2 - \mu_1 + \delta \leq 0 \text{ versus } H_a : \mu_2 - \mu_1 + \delta > 0 \text{ ,.} \qquad (2.4)$$

Example 2.2 Arteriosclerotic Vascular Noninferiority Trial

For the same trial in Example 2.1, suppose we design a noninferiority test, with a margin $\delta = -0.01$ (the determination of δ is a complicated issue and will not be discussed here). The total sample-size can be calculated using (2.3):

$$n = \frac{4(1.96 + 1.28)^2 \left(0.3^2\right)}{\left(0.05 + 0.01\right)^2} = 1050.$$

We can see that the required sample-size is smaller for the noninferiority test than for a superiority test. However, more often we design a noninferiority trial with the belief that two drugs have the same efficacy, that is, $\mu_2 = \mu_1$. In this case, the total sample size is given by

$$n = \frac{4(1.96 + 1.28)^2 \left(0.3^2\right)}{\left(0 + 0.01\right)^2} = 37,791,$$

a dramatic increase, which is practically infeasible to run the noninferiority trial when $\mu_2 = \mu_1$.

2.4   Two-Group Equivalence Trial

The equivalence test for the two parallel groups can be stated as

$$H_0 : |\mu_1 - \mu_2| \geq \delta \quad \text{versus} \quad H_a : |\mu_1 - \mu_2| < \delta, \tag{2.5}$$

where the subscripts 1 and 2 refer to the test and reference groups, respectively. If the null hypothesis is rejected, then we conclude that the test drug and the reference drug are equivalent.

For a large sample-size, the null hypothesis is rejected if

$$T_1 = \frac{\delta - |\bar{x}_1 - \bar{x}_2|}{\sigma \sqrt{\frac{1}{n_1} + \frac{1}{n_2}}} > z_{1-\alpha} . \tag{2.6}$$

The approximate sample-size is given by (Chow, Shao, and Wang, 2003):

$$n_2 = \frac{\left(z_{1-\alpha} + z_{1-\beta/2}\right)^2 \sigma^2 \left(1 + 1/r\right)}{\left(|\varepsilon| - \delta\right)^2}, \tag{2.7}$$

where $r = n_1/n_2$.

Example 2.3 Equivalence LDL Trial

For the LDL trial in Example 2.1, assuming the treatment difference $\varepsilon = 0.01$, $\sigma = 0.3$, and an equivalence margin of $\delta = 0.05$, the sample-size per group for a balanced design ($r = 1$) can be calculated using (2.7) with 90% power at $\alpha = 0.05$ level:

$$n_2 = \frac{(1.6446 + 1.6446)^2 \left(0.3^2\right) (1 + 1/1)}{(0.01 - 0.05)^2} = 1217.$$

Pharmacokinetics (PK) is the study of the body's absorption, distribution, metabolism, and elimination of a drug. An important outcome of a PK study is the bioavailability of the drug. The bioavailability of a drug is defined as the rate and extent to which the active drug ingredient or therapeutic moiety is absorbed and becomes available at the site of drug action. As bioavailability cannot be easily measured directly, the concentration of drug that reaches the circulating bloodstream is taken as a surrogate. Therefore, bioavailability can be viewed as the concentration of drug that is in the blood. Two drugs are bioequivalent if they have the same bioavailability. There are a number of instances in which trials are conducted to show that two drugs are bioequivalent (Jones and Kenward, 2003): (1) when different formulations of the same drug are to be marketed, for instance, in solid-tablet or liquid-capsule form; (2) when a generic version of an innovator drug is to be marketed; (3) when production of a drug is scaled up, and the new production process needs to be shown to produce drugs of equivalent strength and effectiveness to that of the original process.

At the present time, average bioequivalence (ABE) serves as the current international standard for bioequivalence (BE) testing using a 2×2 crossover design. The PK parameters used for assessing ABE are area under the curve (AUC) and peak concentration (Cmax). The recommended statistical method is the two one-sided tests procedure to determine if the average values for the PK measures determined after administration of the T (test) and R (reference) products were comparable. This approach is termed average bioequivalence (ABE). It is equivalent to the so-called confidence interval method, which involves the calculation of a 90% confidence interval for the ratio of the averages (population geometric means) of the measures for the T and R products. To establish BE, the calculated confidence interval should fall within a BE limit, usually $80\% - 125\%$ for the ratio of the product averages. The 1992 guidance has also provided specific recommendations for logarithmic transformation of PK data, methods to evaluate sequence effects, and methods to evaluate outlier data.

In practice, people also use parallel designs and the 90% confidence interval for nontransformed data. To establish BE, the calculated confidence interval should fall within a BE limit, usually $80\% - 120\%$ for the difference of the product averages.

The hypothesis for ABE in a 2×2 crossover design with log-transformed data can be written as

$$H_{01} : \mu_T - \mu_R \leq -\ln 1.25,$$
$$H_{02} : \mu_T - \mu_R \geq \ln 1.25.$$

The asymptotic power is given by (Chow, Shao, and Wang, 2003)

$$n = \frac{\left(z_{1-\alpha} + z_{1-\beta/2}\right)^2 \sigma_{1,1}^2}{2\left(\ln 1.25 - |\varepsilon|\right)^2},$$

where the variance for the intrasubject comparison is estimated using

$$\hat{\sigma}_{1,1}^2 = \frac{1}{n_1 + n_2 - 2} \sum_{j=1}^{2} \sum_{i=1}^{n_j} \left(y_{i1j} - y_{i2j} - \bar{y}_{1j} + \bar{y}_{2j}\right)^2,$$

where y_{ikj} is the log-transformed PK measure from the ith subject in the jth sequence at the kth dosing period, and $\bar{y}_{kj}$ is the sample mean of the observations in the jth sequence at the kth period.

Example 2.4 Average Bioequivalence Trial

Suppose we are interested in establishing ABE between an inhaled formulation and a subcutaneously injected formulation of a test drug. The PK parameter chosen for this bioequivalence test is a log-transformation of the 24-hour AUC (i.e., the raw data are log-normal). Assuming that the difference between the two formulations in log(AUC) is $\varepsilon = 0.04$ and the standard deviation for the intrasubject comparison is $\sigma_{1,1}^2 = 0.55$ with $\alpha = 0.05$ and $\beta = 0.2$, the sample-size per sequence is given by

$$n = \frac{(1.96 + 0.84)^2 (0.55)^2}{2 (0.223 - 0.04)^2} = 36.$$

2.5   Trial with Any Number of Groups

Multigroup trials are often used for dose-finding studies. A commonly used and conservative approach is to compare each active dose to the control using Dunnett's test or a stepwise test. As pointed out by Stewart and Ruberg (2000), the contrast will detect certain expected dose-response features without forcing those expected features into the analysis model. Commonly used contrast procedures include Dunnett's test (Dunnett, 1955), the regression test of Tukey and Heyse 1985, Ruberg's basin contrast (Ruberg, 1998), Williams's test (Williams, 1971, 1972), and the Cochran-Armitage test (Cochran, 1954; Amitage, 1955).

In multiple-arm trials, a general one-sided hypothesis testing problem can be stated as a contrast test:

$$H_0 : \sum_{i=1}^{k} c_i \mu_i - \delta \leq 0; \text{ vs. } H_a : \sum_{i=1}^{k} c_i \mu_i - \delta = \varepsilon > 0, \qquad (2.8)$$

where μ_i can be the mean, proportion, or hazard rate for the ith group depending on the study endpoint, and ε is a constant.

A test statistic can be defined as

$$T = \frac{\sum_{i=1}^{k} c_i \hat{u}_i - \delta}{\sqrt{var_{\varepsilon=0}(\sum_{i=1}^{k} c_i \hat{u}_i - \delta)}} \sim N(\frac{n\varepsilon}{\theta_o}, \frac{\theta_a^2}{\theta_o^2}) \text{ for larger sample size,} \qquad (2.9)$$

where $\hat{u}_i$ is the maximum likelihood estimate of μ_i and the contrast coefficient c_i satisfies the equation $\sum_{i=1}^{k} c_i = 0$ ($c_1 = 1$ for a single-arm trial). Without losing generality, assume that $c_i \mu_i > 0$ indicates efficacy; then, for a superiority design, $\delta \geq 0$, and for a noninferiority design, $\delta < 0$. Note that ε is the treatment difference subtracted from the noninferior/superiority margin δ.

When $\delta = 0$, ε is simply the treatment difference.

$$\varepsilon = \sum_{i=1}^{k} c_i \mu_i - \delta, \tag{2.10}$$

and

$$\begin{cases} \theta_o^2 = \sigma_o^2 \sum_{i=1}^{k} \frac{c_i^2}{f_i} \\ \theta_a^2 = \sum_{i=1}^{k} \frac{c_i^2 \sigma_i^2}{f_i} \end{cases}, \tag{2.11}$$

where n_i is the sample-size for the ith arm, $f_i = \frac{n_i}{n}$ is the size fraction, $n = \sum_{i=0}^{k} n_i$, σ_o^2 is the variance of the response under H_0, and σ_i^2 is the variance under H_a for the ith arm.

Note that if $\delta = 0$ and H_0 defined by (2.8) is rejected for some $\{c_i\}$ satisfying $\sum_{i=1}^{k} c_i = 0$, then there is a difference among μ_i $(i = 1, \ldots, k)$. Under the null hypothesis, the test statistic T follows the standard normal distribution. The power considering heterogeneity of variances can be obtained:

$$\text{power} = \Phi\left(\frac{\varepsilon \sqrt{n} - \theta_o z_{1-\alpha}}{\theta_a}\right). \tag{2.12}$$

Similarly to (2.2), the total sample-size with the heterogeneous variances is given by

$$n = \frac{(z_{1-a}\theta_o + z_{1-\beta}\theta_a)^2}{\varepsilon^2}. \tag{2.13}$$

Equations (2.11) through (2.13) are applicable to any k-arm design ($k \geq 1$). The asymptotic variance σ_i^2 in (2.11) is given in Table 2.1.

It can be seen that (2.12) and (2.13) have included the common one-arm and two-arm superiority and noninferiority designs as special cases: for a one-arm design, $c_1 = 1$, and for a two-arm design, $c_1 = -1$ and $c_2 = 1$.

There are two criteria that need to be considered when selecting contrasts: (1) The selected contrasts must lead to a clinically meaningful hypothesis test, and (2) the selected contrasts should provide the most powerful test statistic after criterion 1.

To use a contrast test, the selection of contrasts should be practically meaningful. If one is interested in a treatment difference among any groups, then any contrasts can be applied. If one is only interested in the comparison between dose-level 1 and other dose levels, then one should make the contrast for dose-level 1 have a different sign from that of the contrasts for other dose groups. Otherwise, efficacy may not be concluded even when the null hypothesis H_0 is rejected, because the rejection of H_0 could be due simply to the opposite effects (some positive and some negative) of different dose levels of the test drug.

Three examples (all modified from the actual trials) will be used to demonstrate the utility of the proposed method for clinical trial designs. The first example is a multiple-arm trial with a continuous endpoint. In the second example, both superiority and noninferiority designs are considered for a multiple-arm trial with a binary endpoint. The third example is an application of the proposed method for designing a multiple-arm trial with a survival endpoint, where different sets of contrasts and balanced, as well as unbalanced, designs are compared. For convenience, the SAS macro for sample-size calculation is provided.

Example 2.5 Dose-Response Trial with Continuous Endpoint

In a phase-II asthma study, a design with 4 dose groups (0 mg, 20 mg, 40 mg, and 60 mg) of the test drug is proposed. The primary efficacy endpoint is the percent change from baseline in forced expiratory volume in the first second (FEV1). From previous studies, it has been estimated that there will be 5%, 12%, 13%, and 14% improvements over baseline for the control, 20 mg, 40 mg, and 60 mg groups, respectively, and a homogeneous standard deviation of $\sigma = 22\%$ for the FEV1 change from baseline. To be consistent with the response shape, let the contrast $c_i = 100(\mu_i - \frac{1}{4}\sum_{i=1}^{4}\mu_i)$, i.e., $c_1 = -6$, $c_2 = 1$, $c_3 = 2$, $c_4 = 3$, where μ_i is the estimated FEV1 improvement in the ith group. It can be seen that any set of contrasts with multiples of the above $\{c_i\}$ will lead to the same sample-size. Thus it can be obtained that $\varepsilon = \sum_{i=1}^{4} c_i\mu_i = 50\%$. Using a balanced design ($f_i = 1/4$) with a one-sided $\alpha = 0.05$, the sample-size required to detect a true difference of $\varepsilon = 0.5$ with 80% power is given by

$$
n = \left[\frac{(z_{1-\alpha} + z_{1-\beta})\sigma}{\varepsilon}\right]^2 \sum_{i=1}^{4} \frac{c_i^2}{f_i}
$$
$$
= \left[\frac{(1.645 + 0.842)(0.22)}{0.50}\right]^2 4((-6)^2 + 1^2 + 2^2 + 3^2)
$$
$$
= 240.
$$

Thus, a total sample-size of 240 is required for the trial.

Example 2.6 Dose-Response Trial with Binary Endpoint

A trial is to be designed for patients with acute ischemic stroke of recent onset. The composite endpoint (death and myocardial infarction [MI]) is the primary endpoint. There are four dose levels planned with event rates of 14%, 13%, 12%, and 11%, respectively. The first group is the active control group (14% event rate). The trial is interested in both superiority and noninferiority tests comparing the test drug to the active control. Notice that there is no need for multiplicity adjustment for the two tests because of the closed-set test procedure. The comparisons are made between the active control and the test groups; therefore, the contrast for the active control should have a different sign than the contrasts for the test groups. Let $c_1 = -6$, $c_2 = 1$, $c_3 = 2$, and $c_4 = 3$. It is assumed that the noninferiority margin for the event rate is $\delta = 0.5\%$, and the event rate is $p_o = 0.14$ under the null hypothesis. Because it is a noninferiority design and the noninferiority margin is usually defined based on a two-arm design, to make this noninferiority margin usable in the multiple-arm design, the contrasts need to be rescaled to match the two-arm design, i.e., set the contrast for the control group $c_1 = -1$. The final contrasts used in the trial are given by $\{c_1 = -1,\ c_2 = \frac{1}{6},\ c_3 = \frac{1}{3},\ c_4 = \frac{1}{2}\}$. Based on this information, it can be obtained that $\varepsilon = \sum_{i=1}^{k} c_i p_i - \delta = -0.02333 - 0.005 = -0.02833$, where p_i is the estimated event rate in the ith group. Using a balanced design ($f_i = 1/4$), the two key parameters, θ_o^2 and θ_a^2, can be calculated as follows:

$$\begin{cases} \theta_o^2 = p_o(1 - p_o) \sum_{i=1}^{k} \frac{c_i^2}{f_i} = 0.6689 \\ \theta_a^2 = \sum_{i=1}^{k} \frac{c_i^2\, p_i(1-p_i)}{f_i} = 0.639 \end{cases}.$$

Using a one-sided $\alpha = 0.025$ and a power of 90%, the total sample-size required for the noninferiority test is given by

$$\begin{aligned} n &= \left[\frac{(z_{1-\alpha}\theta_o + z_{1-\beta}\theta_a)}{\varepsilon} \right]^2 \\ &= \left[\frac{(1.96\sqrt{0.6689} + 1.2815\sqrt{0.639})}{-0.02833} \right]^2 \\ &= 8,600. \end{aligned}$$

Thus a total sample-size of 8,600 patients is required for the noninferiority test. With 8,600 patients, the power for the superiority test ($\delta = 0,\varepsilon = 0.0233$) is 76.5%, which is calculated as follows:

$$\begin{aligned} \text{power} &= \Phi_o \left(\frac{\varepsilon\sqrt{n} - \theta_o z_{1-\alpha}}{\theta_a} \right) \\ &= \Phi_o \left(\frac{0.0233\sqrt{8600} - 1.96\sqrt{0.6689}}{\sqrt{0.639}} \right) \\ &= \Phi_o (0.6977) = 76\%. \end{aligned}$$

An interesting note is that the Cochran-Armitage linear trend test is a special case of the contrast test in which the contrast $c_i = d_i - \bar{d}$, where d_i is the ith dose and $\bar{d}$ is the average dose.

Example 2.7 Two-Group Design with Survival Endpoint

Let λ_i be the population hazard rate for group i. The contrast test for multiple survival curves can be written as $H_0 : \sum_{i=0}^{k} c_i \lambda_i \leq 0$. For two-group design, we can choose $c_1 = 1$ and $c_2 = -1$. Suppose that, in this phase-III oncology trial, the objective is to determine if there is treatment effect with time-to-progression as the primary endpoint. Patient enrollment duration is estimated to be $T_0 = 9$ months and the total trial duration is $T_s = 16$ months. Under the exponential survival distribution, $\lambda = \frac{\ln 2}{T_{Median}}$. The estimated median times are 15.1 months (hazard rate 0.0459/month) and 22 months (hazard rate 0.0315/month) for the control and test groups, respectively. Thus, the treatment difference is given by $\varepsilon = \sum_{i=0}^{k} c_i \lambda_i = 0.0459 - 0.0315 = 0.014\,4$. The variances are given by

$$\sigma_1^2 = 0.0459^2 \left(1 - \frac{e^{0.0459 \times 9} - 1}{(9)0.0459 e^{0.0459 \times 16}} \right)^{-1} = 0.0052$$

$$\sigma_2^2 = 0.0315^2 \left(1 - \frac{e^{0.0315 \times 9} - 1}{(9)0.0315 e^{0.0315 \times 16}} \right)^{-1} = 0.0033.$$

For a balanced design with sample size fraction $f_1 = f_2 = 0.5$, we have

$$\begin{cases} \theta_o^2 = \sigma_1^2 \sum_{i=1}^{k} \frac{c_i^2}{f_i} = 0.0052(\frac{2}{0.5}) = 0.020\,8 \\ \theta_a^2 = \sum_{i=1}^{k} \frac{c_i^2 \sigma_i^2}{f_i} = \frac{0.0052 + 0.0033}{0.5} = 0.017 \end{cases} .$$

Using a one-sided $\alpha = 0.025$ and a power of 90%, the total sample-size required for the survival endpoint test is given by

$$n = \left[\frac{(1.96\sqrt{0.020\,8} + 1.2815\sqrt{0.017})}{0.014\,4} \right]^2 = 974.$$

Note that some software packages, e.g., ExpDesign Studio 5.0, use the approximation in the two-group survival design with the common variance $\frac{\sigma_1^2 + \sigma_2^2}{2}$, which will give sample size of about 860.

Using the patient-event relationship,

$$D = \begin{cases} \frac{n}{T_0} \left(T - \frac{1}{\lambda} + \frac{1}{\lambda} e^{-\lambda T} \right), & T \leq T_0 \\ \frac{n}{T_0} \left(T_0 - \frac{1}{\lambda} \left(e^{\lambda T_0} - 1 \right) e^{-\lambda T} \right), & T > T_0, \end{cases}$$

we can calculate the number of events required in the control and test groups: 395 and 294, or a total of 689 events. This number of events is based on the recruitment duration $T_s = 9$ months and study duration $T = 16$ months. If the study duration is longer or the recruitment duration shorter, the number of events will be more and the power will be higher.

Table 2.2: Critical Value c_α for Classical Dunnett Test

	K, Number of Active Arms						
N/Arm	1	2	3	4	5	6	7
15	2.050	2.335	2.492	2.602	2.685	2.753	2.803
50	1.983	2.246	2.389	2.487	2.558	2.614	2.668
300	1.960	2.221	2.356	2.445	2.513	2.576	2.626

Note: 1,000,000 runs per scenario, equal sample size.

2.6 Multigroup Dose-Finding Trial

The Dunnett test is used when there are K active arms and one common control arm. There are K multiple tests; each test consists of the comparison between the active and the control with the null hypotheses:

$$H_i : \mu_i = \mu_0, \ i = 1, \ldots, K. \tag{2.14}$$

Dunnett's test is based on K-variate normal distribution:

$$\boldsymbol{T} \sim \boldsymbol{N}\left(\boldsymbol{\mu}, \boldsymbol{\Sigma}\right). \tag{2.15}$$

Dunnett used an equal critical value c_α for all K tests such that the rejection probability under the global null hypothesis H_G is α. This is equivalent to using the maximum test statistic among all T_i $(i = 1, \ldots K)$ to determine the c_α because (1) if we use this c_α to test all H_i, the type-I error rate under global H_G will be α since, as long as any H_i is rejected, the one with maximum test statistic T is rejected, (2) if H_i with maximum test statistic T is not rejected, then no H_i should be rejected.

Therefore, to control the familywise type-I error for Dunnett's test with larger sample size, Chang proved (2014) the distribution (c.d.f.) of the maximum test statistic T to be

$$F_T\left(t\right) = \int_{-\infty}^{\infty} \left[\Phi\left(z\right)\right]^K \phi\left(\sqrt{2}t - z\right) dz. \tag{2.16}$$

Table 2.2 shows critical value for the maximum Dunnett Test for $\alpha = 0.025$ and 0.05.

We have provided the R function for Dunnett's test in the Appendix B. The typical R code to invoke the function is presented as follows:

```
## Determine critical value Zalpha for alpha (power) =0.025 ##
ns=c(288,288,288); us=c(0,0,0); sigmas=c(2,2,2)
powerDunnett(n0=288,u0=0,sigma0=2,nArms=3,cAlpha=2.361,nSims=10000)
## Determine Power ##
ns=c(288,288,288); us=c(0.3,0.4,0.5); sigmas=c(2,2,2)
powerDunnett(n0=288,u0=0,sigma0=2,nArms=3,cAlpha=2.361,nSims=10000)
```

Commonly used contrast procedures include Dunnett's test (Dunnett, 1955).

2.7   Summary and Discussion

In this chapter, we reviewed commonly used classical trial design methods. The methods derived from a contrast test can be used for power and sample-size calculations for k-arm trials ($k \geq 1$). They can be used for superiority or noninferiority designs with continuous, binary, or survival endpoints. The selection of contrasts is critical. The selected contrasts must lead to a clinically meaningful hypothesis test and should lead to a powerful test statistic. In a phase-II clinical trial, we often want to compare multiple active arms to a common control. In this case, Dunnett's test is the most common test to use because it controls the familywise error strongly.

It is important to remember that the power very much relies on the assumption of the estimated effect size at the time of study design. It is even more critical to fully understand these three different concepts about effect size: true size, estimated size, and minimum meaningful effect size, and their impacts on trial design. Last but not least, trial design involves many different aspects of medical/scientific, statistical, commercial, regulatory, and operational, data management functions. A statistician cannot view the achievement of a design with the greatest power or smallest sample-size as the ultimate goal. Further, a trial design cannot be viewed as an isolated task. Instead, drug development should be viewed as an integrated process in which a sequence of decisions are made. We will discuss more on this throughout the book.

Chapter 3

Two-Stage Adaptive Confirmatory Design Method

3.1 General Formulation

In this chapter, we will discuss three methods for two-stage adaptive design methods. The methods are differentiated in terms of the test statistics defined at each stage, while the test statistic is evidence against the null hypothesis in terms of cumulative information (data). The three methods are constructed based on three different ways to combine the so-called stagewise p-values: (1) the sum of p-values (MSP), (2) the product of p-values (MPP), and (3) the inverse-normal p-values (MINP). The MINP is a generalization of the test statistics used in the classical group sequential design. The operating characteristics of MPP and MINP are very similar. The methods are very general, meaning that they can be applied to broad adaptations and any number of stages in the adaptive trials. However, we will focus on two-stage designs and provide the closed forms for determination of stopping boundaries. We will design different group sequential trials using these methods, while the applications of the methods to other types of adaptive designs will be discussed later. Power and sample-size calculations for the adaptive designs are based on computer simulations.

Suppose, in a two-group parallel design trial, that the objective is to test the treatment difference

$$H_0 : \mu_1 = \mu_2 \text{ versus } H_a : \mu_1 > \mu_2. \tag{3.1}$$

A one-sided test is always used in this book unless otherwise specified. An adaptive trial usually consists of several stages; at each stage a decision needs to made to reject or accept the null hypothesis, or continue the trial on the next stage to collect more data, or other adaptations.

The test statistic at the kth stage is denoted by T_k, which is constructed based on cumulative data at the time of analysis. A convenient way to combine the data from different stages is to combine p_i $(i = 1, 2)$, the p-value from the subsample obtained at the ith stage. For a normal endpoint, the stagewise

p-value is $p_i = 1 - \Phi(z_i)$, where z_i is z-score calculated based on the subsample obtained at the ith stage.

For group sequential design, the stopping rules at the first stage are

$$\begin{cases} \text{Reject } H_0 \text{ (stop for efficacy) if } T_1 \le \alpha_1, \\ \text{Accept } H_0 \text{ (stop for futility) if } T_1 > \beta_1, \\ \text{Continue with adaptations} \quad \text{if } \alpha_1 < T_1 \le \beta_1, \end{cases} \quad (3.2)$$

where $0 \le \alpha_1 < \beta_1 \le 1$.

The stopping rules at the second stage are

$$\begin{cases} \text{Stop for efficacy} \ \ \text{if } T_1 \le \alpha_2, \\ \text{Stop for futility} \ \ \text{if } T_1 > \alpha_2. \end{cases} \quad (3.3)$$

For convenience, α_k and β_k are called the efficacy and futility boundaries, respectively.

To reach the second stage, a trial has to pass the first stage. Therefore, the probability of rejecting the null hypothesis H_0 or, simply, the rejection probability at the second stage is given by

$$\Pr(\alpha_1 < T_1 < \beta_1, T_k < \alpha_2) = \int_{\alpha_1}^{\beta_1} \int_{-\infty}^{\alpha_2} f_{T_1 T_2}(t_1, t_2) \, dt_2 dt_1, \quad (3.4)$$

where $f_{T_1 T_2}$ is the joint probability density function (p.d.f.) p.d.f. of T_1 and T_2.

When the futility boundary $\beta_1 = 1$, futility stopping is impossible. In this case, the efficacy boundary at the second stage α_2 is determined by formulation $\alpha_1 + \Pr(\alpha_1 < T_1 < 1, T_k < \alpha_2) = \alpha$. In comparison with the efficacy boundary α_2^* when there is a futility boundary β_1, it is obvious that $\Pr(\alpha_1 < T_1 < \beta_1, T_k < \alpha_2) = \Pr(\alpha_1 < T_1, T_k < \alpha_2^*)$. It follows that $\alpha_2^* \le \alpha_2$. However, in current practice, the futility boundary β_1 may not be followed by the pharmaceutical industry (nonbinding futility boundary); therefore, the FDA will not accept the α_2^* for the phase-III studies. Instead, the nonbinding futility boundary α_2 is suggested. This is the so-called FDA's *nonbinding futility rule*.

3.2 Method Based on Sum of p-Values

Chang (2006a) proposed an adaptive design method, in which the test statistic is defined as the sum of the stagewise p-values. This method is referred to as MSP and the test statistic at the kth stage is defined as

$$T_k = \Sigma_{i=1}^{k} p_i, \ \ k = 1, \ldots, K. \quad (3.5)$$

Table 3.1: Stopping Boundaries with MSP

α_1	0.0000	0.00250	0.0050	0.0100	0.0150	0.0200
α_2	0.22361	0.21463	0.20500	0.18321	0.15642	0.12000

Note: One-sided $\alpha = 0.025$.

Let π_1 and π_2 be the type-I errors spent (i.e., the probability of false rejection allowed) at the first and second stages, respectively. Under the nonbinding futility rule $(\beta_1 = \alpha_2)$, the stopping boundaries α_1 and α_2 must satisfy the following equations:

$$\begin{cases} \pi_1 = \alpha_1 \\ \pi_2 = \frac{1}{2}(\alpha_2 - \alpha_1)^2. \end{cases} \tag{3.6}$$

Since $\pi_1 + \pi_2 = \alpha$, the stopping boundaries can be written as

$$\begin{cases} \alpha_1 = \pi_1, \\ \alpha_2 = \sqrt{2(\alpha - \pi_1)} + \pi_1. \end{cases} \tag{3.7}$$

As soon as we decide the significant level α and π_1, we can determine the stopping boundaries α_1 and α_2 using (3.7); see numerical examples in Table 3.1.

Example 3.1 Group Sequential Design for Asthma Study with MSP

Asthma is a chronic disease characterized by airway inflammation. Those affected with the disease experience asthmatic episodes when their airways narrow due to inflammation and they have difficulty breathing. According to the US centers for Disease Control and Prevention (CDC), about 1 in 12 people (about 25 million) have asthma, and the numbers are increasing every year. About 1 in 2 people (about 12 million) with asthma had an asthma attack in 2008, but many asthma attacks could have been prevented. The number of people diagnosed with asthma grew by 4.3 million from 2001 to 2009. Asthma was linked to 3,447 deaths in 2007. Asthma costs in the US grew from about \$53 billion in 2002 to about \$56 billion in 2007, about a 6% increase. Greater access to medical care is needed for the growing number of people with asthma.

In a phase-III asthma study with 2 dose groups (control and test), the primary efficacy endpoint is the percent change from baseline in FEV1. The estimated FEV1 improvement from baseline is 5% and 12% for the control and active groups, respectively, with a common standard deviation of $\sigma = 22\%$. Based on a large sample assumption, the sample-size for a fixed design is 208 per group, which has 90% power to detect the difference at a one-sided alpha $= 0.025$. Using MSP, an interim analysis is planned based on the response assessments of 115 (50%) patients. To design a group sequential trial, we chose

Table 3.2: Operating Characteristics of a GSD with MSP

Simulation condition	ESP	FSP	$\bar{N}$	N_{max}	Power (alpha)
Classical	0	0	416	416	0.90
GSD (H_a)	0.56	0	347	480	0.90
GSD (H_0)	0.01	0	447	480	(0.025)

to stop; boundaries at the first stage: $\alpha_1 = \pi_1 = 0.01$, then from Table 3.1 or formulation (3.7), we can obtain $\alpha_2 = 0.18321$.

To calculate the power and expected sample size under the alternative hypothesis with FEV1 improvement $\mu_0 = 0.05$ and $\mu_1 = 0.12$ for the control and test groups, respectively, we can invoke the R function as follows:

TwoStageGSDwithNormalEndpoint(u0=0.05,u1=0.12,sigma0=0.22,sigma1=0.22,
n0Stg1=120,n1Stg1=120,n0Stg2=120,n1Stg2=120,alpha1=0.01,beta1=1,
alpha2=0.18321,method="MSP")

Similarly, we can calculate the expected sample size when the null hypothesis is true ($\mu_0 = \mu_1 = 0.05$) by invoking the same R function with the following line of code:

TwoStageGSDwithNormalEndpoint(u0=0.05,u1=0.05,sigma0=0.22,sigma1=0.22,
n0Stg1=120,n1Stg1=120,n0Stg2=120,n1Stg2=120,alpha1=0.01,beta1=1,
alpha2=0.18321, method="MSP")

The simulation results are summarized in Table 3.2.

From Table 3.2, we can see that the GSD has a smaller expected sample-size ($\bar{N}$) under H_a (347) than the classical design (416). If the trial stops early, only 240 patients are required. The probability of early efficacy stopping is 56%. However, the group sequential design has a larger maximum sample-size (480) than the classical design does (416). The sample size under H_0 is also larger with GSD (447) than the classical design (416). We will discuss later how to reduce the sample size under H_0 using futility boundaries.

3.3   Method with Product of p-Values

This method is referred to as MPP. The test statistic in this method is based on the product of the stagewise p-values from the subsamples. For two-stage designs, the test statistic is defined as (Bauer and Kohne, 1994)

$$T_k = \Pi_{i=1}^k p_i, \ \ k = 1, 2. \tag{3.8}$$

Under the nonbinding futility rule ($\beta_1 = 1$), the α spent at the two stages are given by

Table 3.3: Stopping Boundaries α_2 with MPP

α_1	0.001	0.0025	0.005	0.010	0.015	0.020
α_2	0.0035	0.0038	0.0038	0.0033	0.0024	0.0013

Note: One-sided $\alpha = 0.025$.

$$\begin{cases} \pi_1 = \alpha_1, \\ \pi_2 = -\alpha_2 \ln \alpha_1. \end{cases}$$

Since $\pi_1 + \pi_2 = \alpha$, the stopping boundaries can be written as

$$\begin{cases} \alpha_1 = \pi_1, \\ \alpha_2 = \frac{\pi_1 - \alpha}{\ln \pi_1}. \end{cases} \tag{3.9}$$

As soon as we decide α and π_1, we can determine the stopping boundaries α_1 and α_2 using (3.9); see numerical examples in Table 3.3.

It is interesting to know that when $p_1 < \alpha_2$, there is no point in continuing the trial because $p_1 p_2 < p_1 < \alpha_2$ and efficacy should be claimed. Therefore it is suggested that we should choose $\beta_1 > \alpha_1 > \alpha_2$.

Example 3.2 Group Sequential Design for Asthma Study with MPP

For the same asthma trial in Example 3.1, we use MPP this time instead of MSP by invoking the R function with the following lines of code for H_a and H_0, respectively:

```
TwoStageGSDwithNormalEndpoint(u0=0.05,u1=0.12,sigma0=0.22,sigma1=0.22,
n0Stg1=113,n1Stg1=113,n0Stg2=113,n1Stg2=113,alpha1=0.01,beta1=1,
alpha2=0.0033,method="MPP")
TwoStageGSDwithNormalEndpoint(u0=0.05,u1=0.05,sigma0=0.22,sigma1=0.22,
n0Stg1=113,n1Stg1=113,n0Stg2=113,n1Stg2=113,alpha1=0.01,beta1=1,
alpha2=0.0033,method="MPP")
```

We can see from the simulation results (Table 3.4) that this GSD with MPP is similar to but slightly better in terms of sample size than previous GSD with MSP.

Table 3.4: Operating Characteristics of a GSD with MPP

Simulation condition	ESP	FSP	$\bar{N}$	N_{max}	Power (alpha)
Classical	0	0	416	416	0.90
GSD (H_a)	0.53	0	333	452	0.90
GSD (H_0)	0.01	0	450	452	(0.025)

3.4   Method with Inverse-Normal p-Values

Lehmacher and Wassmer (1999) proposed the test statistic at the kth stage that results from the inverse-normal method of combining independent stage-wise p-values:

$$Z_k = \sum_{i=1}^{k} w_{ki} \Phi^{-1}(1-p_i), \qquad (3.10)$$

where the weights satisfy the equality $\sum_{i=1}^{k} w_{ki}^2 = 1$, and Φ^{-1} is the inverse function of Φ, the standard normal c.d.f. Under the null hypothesis, the stagewise p_i is usually uniformly distributed over [0,1]. The random variables $z_{1-p_i} = \Phi^{-1}(1-p_i)$ and Z_k have the standard normal distribution. MINP is a generalization of classical GSD (details will be provided later).

To be consistent with MSP and MPP, we transform the test statistic Z_k to the p-scale, i.e.,

$$T_k = 1 - \Phi\left(\sum_{i=1}^{k} w_{ki} \Phi^{-1}(1-p_i)\right). \qquad (3.11)$$

With (3.11), the stopping boundary is on the p-scale and easy to compare with other methods regarding operating characteristics.

When the test statistic defined by (3.11) is used, the classical group sequential boundaries are valid regardless of the timing and sample-size adjustment that may be based on the observed data at the previous stages. Note that under the null hypothesis, p_i is usually uniformly distributed over [0,1] and hence $z_{1-p_i} = \Phi^{-1}(1-p_i)$ has the standard normal distribution. The Lehmacher-Wassmer method provides a broad method for different endpoints as long as the p-value under the null hypothesis is stochastically larger than or equal to the p-value that is uniformly distributed over [0,1].

Examples of stopping boundaries for a two-stage design with weights, $w_1^2 = \frac{n_1}{n_1+n_2}$, are presented in Table 3.5.

Table 3.5: Stopping Boundaries α_2 with Equal Weights

w_1^2	α_1					
	0.0000	0.0025	0.0050	0.0100	0.0150	0.0200
1/4	0.0250	0.0233	0.0212	0.0168	0.0120	0.0064
1/3	0.0250	0.0235	0.0217	0.0174	0.0126	0.0071
1/2	0.0250	0.0240	0.0225	0.0188	0.0143	0.0086
3/4	0.0250	0.0247	0.0241	0.0219	0.0184	0.0130

Note: One-sided $\alpha = 0.025$ and 1,000,000 simulation runs.

Note that w_1^2 don't have to be equal to $\frac{n_1}{n_1+n_2}$. If $w_1^2 \neq \frac{n_1}{n_1+n_2}$, the stopping boundaries in Table 3.5 cannot be used, but can use simulations to determine them.

In classical group sequential design (GSD), the stopping boundaries are usually specified using a function of stage k. The commonly used such functions are Pocock and O'Brien-Fleming boundary functions. Wang and Tsiatis (1987) proposed a family of two-sided tests with a shape parameter Δ, which includes Pocock's and O'Brien-Fleming's boundary functions as special cases. Because W-T boundaries are based on the z-scale, for consistency, we can convert them to p-scale. The W-T boundary on p-scale is given by

$$a_k = 1 - \Phi \left(\alpha_K \, \tau_k^{\Delta-1/2} \right), \tag{3.12}$$

where $\tau_k = \frac{k}{K}$ or $\tau_k = \frac{n_k}{N_K}$ (information time), and α_K is the stopping boundary at the final stage and a function of the number of stages K, α,and Δ.

Let n_i = stagewise sample-size per group at stage i and $N_k = \Sigma_{i=1}^k n_i$ be the cumulative sample-size at stage k and the information fraction (not information time!). If we choose $w_{ki} = \sqrt{\frac{n_i}{N_k}}$, then the MINP is consistent with the classical group sequential design.

Example 3.3: Group Sequential Design for Asthma Study with MINP

For the same asthma trial in Example 3.1, we use MINP by invoking the same R function with the following lines of code for H_a and H_0, respectively:

```
TwoStageGSDwithNormalEndpoint(u0=0.05,u1=0.12,sigma0=0.22,sigma1=0.22,
n0Stg1=110,n1Stg1=110,n0Stg2=110,n1Stg2=110,alpha1=0.01,beta1=1,
alpha2=0.0188,w1squared=0.5,method="MINP")
TwoStageGSDwithNormalEndpoint(u0=0.05,u1=0.05,sigma0=0.22,sigma1=0.22,
n0Stg1=110,n1Stg1=110,n0Stg2=110,n1Stg2=110,alpha1=0.01,beta1=1,
alpha2=0.0188,w1squared=0.5,method="MINP")
```

We can see from the simulation results in Table 3.6 that this GSD with MINP is similar to the results from MPP.

A commonly used stopping boundary is the so-called O'Brien-Fleming boundaries, which on p-scale are $\alpha_1 = 0.0026$, $\alpha_2 = 0.024$ for a one-sided

Table 3.6: Operating Characteristics of a GSD with MINP

Simulation condition	ESP	FSP	$\bar{N}$	N_{max}	Power (alpha)
Classical	0	0	416	416	0.90
GSD (H_a)	0.51	0	328	440	0.90
GSD (H_0)	0.01	0	438	440	(0.025)

Table 3.7: Operating Characteristics of O'Brien-Fleming GSD

Simulation condition	ESP	FSP	$\bar{N}$	N_{max}	Power (alpha)
Classical	0	0	416	416	0.90
GSD (H_a)	0.31	0	354	420	0.90
GSD (H_0)	0.01	0	419	420	(0.025)

significance level of 0.025. To see how this change of efficacy stopping boundary will affect the operating characteristics of the GSD, we invoke R function with the following lines of code for the conditions H_a and H_0, respectively:

```
TwoStageGSDwithNormalEndpoint(u0=0.05,u1=0.12,sigma0=0.22,sigma1=0.22,
n0Stg1=105,n1Stg1=105,n0Stg2=105,n1Stg2=105,alpha1=0.0026,beta1=1,
alpha2=0.024,w1squared=0.5,method="MINP")
TwoStageGSDwithNormalEndpoint(u0=0.05,u1=0.05,sigma0=0.22,sigma1=0.22,
n0Stg1=105,n1Stg1=105,n0Stg2=105,n1Stg2=105,alpha1=0.0026,beta1=1,
alpha2=0.024,w1squared=0.5,method="MINP")
```

Comparing the simulation results in Table 3.6 and Table 3.7, we can see that the O'Brien-Fleming boundary with a smaller type-I error ($\pi_1 = \alpha_1$) at the first stage will reduce the probability of early efficacy stopping (ESP1 = 0.51 versus 0.31) and increase the expected sample size under H_a, but reduce the maximum sample size from 440 to 420 under H_a and the expected sample size from 438 to 419 under H_0. The effect of the futility boundary will be investigated later.

3.5   Comparisons of Adaptive Design Methods

Example 3.4 Early Futility Stopping GSD for Asthma Study

We now study the effect of a futility stopping boundary on the operating characteristics of GSD. Again, we use the asthma trial in Example 3.1. We choose the futility boundary $\beta_1 = 0.022$ and the popular O'Brien-Fleming type boundary for efficacy with $\alpha_1 = 0.0026$, and $\alpha_2 = 0.024$ for MINP, $\alpha_2 = 0.2143$ for MSP from (3.7), and $\alpha_2 = 0.0038$ for MPP from (3.9). After invoking the R function with the following lines of code, we obtain the simulation results in Table 3.8. Note that we follow the nonbinding futility rule; thus the futility boundary will not affect the determination of efficacy boundary α_2. We use the following lines of R code to run the simulations:

```
TwoStageGSDwithNormalEndpoint(u0=0.05,u1=0.12,sigma0=0.22,sigma1=0.22,
n0Stg1=124,n1Stg1=124,n0Stg2=105,n1Stg2=105,alpha1=0.0026,
beta1=0.2143,alpha2=0.2143,method="MSP")
TwoStageGSDwithNormalEndpoint(u0=0.05,u1=0.05,sigma0=0.22,sigma1=0.22,
```

Table 3.8: Operating Characteristics of O'Brien-Fleming GSD

Method	α_1	α_2	β_1	$\bar{N}_0$	$\tilde{N}_a$	N_{max}	Power
MSP	0.0026	0.2143	0.2143	292	367	458	0.90
MPP	0.0026	0.0038	0.2143	304	376	470	0.90
MINP	0.0026	0.0240	0.2143	281	369	464	0.90

n0Stg1=124,n1Stg1=124,n0Stg2=105,n1Stg2=105,alpha1=0.0026,
beta1=0.2143,alpha2=0.2143,method="MSP")
TwoStageGSDwithNormalEndpoint(u0=0.05,u1=0.12,sigma0=0.22,sigma1=0.22,
n0Stg1=130,n1Stg1=130,n0Stg2=105,n1Stg2=105,alpha1=0.0026,
beta1=0.2143,alpha2=0.0038,method="MPP")
TwoStageGSDwithNormalEndpoint(u0=0.05,u1=0.05,sigma0=0.22,sigma1=0.22,
n0Stg1=130,n1Stg1=130,n0Stg2=105,n1Stg2=105,alpha1=0.0026,
beta1=0.2143,alpha2=0.0038,method="MPP")
TwoStageGSDwithNormalEndpoint(u0=0.05,u1=0.12,sigma0=0.22,sigma1=0.22,
n0Stg1=116,n1Stg1=116,n0Stg2=116,n1Stg2=116,alpha1=0.0026,
beta1=0.2143,alpha2=0.024,w1squared=0.5,method="MINP")
TwoStageGSDwithNormalEndpoint(u0=0.05,u1=0.05,sigma0=0.22,sigma1=0.22,
n0Stg1=116,n1Stg1=116,n0Stg2=116,n1Stg2=116,alpha1=0.0026,
beta1=0.2143,alpha2=0.024,w1squared=0.5,method="MINP")

The simulation results show that in this case, MSP and MINP provide similar operating characteristics and they are better than MPP. Comparing the MINP results in Table 3.7 and MINP results in Table 3.8, we can see that adding a futility boundary can reduce the expected sample size under H_0, but at the same time increase the maximum sample size.

So far we have studied the GSD for the trial with a normal endpoint. For the binary endpoint, the GSD is similar under larger sample size assumptions, for which the "equivalent standard deviation" is $\sigma_i^* = \sqrt{r_i(1 - r_i)}$, where r_i is the response rate in group i.

Example 3.5 Group Sequential Trial for Acute Coronary Syndromes

Acute coronary syndrome (ACS) refers to any group of symptoms attributed to obstruction of the coronary arteries. Acute coronary syndrome symptoms may include the type of chest pressure that you feel during a heart attack, or pressure in your chest while you're at rest or doing light physical activity (unstable angina). The first sign of acute coronary syndrome can be sudden stopping of your heart (cardiac arrest). Acute coronary syndrome usually occurs as a result of one of three problems: ST elevation myocardial infarction (30%), non-ST elevation myocardial infarction (25%), or unstable angina (38%) (Torres and Moayedi, 2007).

Aggregation of platelets is the pathophysiologic basis of the acute coronary syndromes. EPT, a hypothetical drug candidate, is an inhibitor of the platelet glycoprotein IIb/IIIa receptor, which is involved in platelet aggregation. A phase-III trial is to be designed for patients with acute ischemic stroke of recent onset. The sponsor and investigator want to know if inhibition of platelet aggregation with EPT will have an incremental benefit beyond that of heparin and aspirin in reducing the frequency of adverse outcomes in patients with acute coronary syndromes who did not have persistent ST-segment elevation. The composite endpoint (death or MI) is the primary endpoint and the event rate is estimated to be 14% for the control group and 12% for the test group. Based on a large sample assumption, the sample-size for a fixed design is 5,076 per group, which provides 85% power to detect the difference at one-sided alpha = 0.025.

There was a concern that if the test drug did not work, the sponsor would want to stop earlier with a smaller sample size. For this reason, a two-stage GSD was proposed with the interim analysis to be performed based on 50% patients. We used O'Brien-Fleming efficacy boundaries with $\alpha_1 = 0.0026$, $\alpha_2 = 0.024$, and a futility boundary $\beta_1 = 0.5$. After we tried different sample sizes for the targeted 85% power, we determined that $N_{max} = 5,160$ per group was needed. The operating characteristics are presented in Table 3.9. The GSD required a smaller expected sample size (3,866 and 4,455 under H_0 and H_a, respectively) than the classical design.

Here are the lines of R code that invoke the R function for the simulation results in Table 3.9:

```
TwoStageGSDwithVariousEndpoints(u0=.12,u1=.14,nStg1=2580,nStg2=2580, alpha1=.0026,beta1=0.5,alpha2=.024,method="MINP",w1squared=0.5,
endpoint="binary")
TwoStageGSDwithVariousEndpoints(u0=.14,u1=.14,nStg1=2580,nStg2=2580, alpha1=.0026,beta1=0.5,alpha2=.024,          method="MINP",w1squared=0.5,
endpoint="binary")
```

Example 3.6: Adaptive Design for Oncology Trial

Cancer is a broad group of diseases involving unregulated cell growth. In cancer, cells divide and grow uncontrollably, forming malignant tumors, which may invade nearby parts of the body. The cancer may also spread to more

Table 3.9: GSD Acute Coronary Syndromes with MINP

Scenario	ESP	FSP	$\bar{N}$	N_{max}	Power (alpha)
Classical	0	0	5076	5076	0.85
H_o	0.002	0.500	3866	5160	(0.025)
H_a	0.256	0.017	4455	5160	0.85

distant parts of the body through the lymphatic system or bloodstream. There are over 200 different known cancers that affect humans.

In a two-arm comparative oncology trial, the primary efficacy endpoint is time-to-progression (TTP). The median TTP is estimated to be 8 months (hazard rate = 0.08664) for the control group, and 10.5 months (hazard rate = 0.06601) for the test group. Assume a uniform enrollment with an accrual period of 9 months and a total study duration of 24 months. The log-rank test will be used for the analysis. An exponential survival distribution is assumed for the purpose of sample-size calculation. The classical design requires a sample-size of 375 subjects per group for 90% power at 0.025 significance level.

We design the trial with one interim analysis when 40% of patients have been enrolled. The interim analysis for efficacy is planned based on TTP, but it does not allow for futility stopping. Using GSD with MINP and O'Brien-Fleming stopping boundaries, $\alpha_1 = 0.0026$, $\beta_1 = 1$, and $\alpha_2 = 0.024$.

Here are the lines of R code that invoke the R function for the simulation results in Table 3.10:

```
TwoStageGSDwithVariousEndpoints(u0=0.06601,u1=0.08664,nStg1=190,
nStg2=190,alpha1=.0026,beta1=1,alpha2=.024,method="MINP",
w1squared=0.5,endpoint="survival")
TwoStageGSDwithVariousEndpoints(u0=0.08664,u1=0.08664,nStg1=190,
nStg2=190,alpha1=.0026,beta1=1,alpha2=.024,method="MINP",
w1squared=0.5,endpoint="survival")
```

We now summarize the simulation outputs for three different scenarios in Table 3.10. We see that the expected sample size reduces from 375 per group for the classical design to 321 per group for the GSD. The cost for the oncology trial is about 100,000 USD per patient.

Example 3.7: Adaptive Design for Oncology NI Trial

Suppose we want to design a noninferiority trial in Example 3.6 instead of a superiority trial. The noninferiority margin is determined to be $NId = 0.005$ in terms of hazard rate. We invoke the following code for the simulations:

Table 3.10: GSD Acute Coronary Syndromes with MINP

Scenario	ESP	FSP	$\bar{N}$	N_{max}	Power (alpha)
Classical	0	0	375	375	0.90
H_o	0.003	0	379	380	(0.025)
H_a	0.311	0	321	380	0.90

Table 3.11: GSD Acute Coronary Syndromes with MINP

Scenario	ESP	FSP	$\bar{N}$	N_{max}	Power (alpha)
Classical	0	0	375	375	0.90
H_o	0.003	0	246	246	(0.025)
H_a	0.308	0	208	246	0.90

TwoStageGSDwithVariousEndpoints(u0=0.06601,u1=0.08664,nStg1=123,
nStg2=123,alpha1=0.0026,beta1=1,alpha2=0.024,method="MINP",
w1squared=0.5,endpoint="survival",NId=0.005)
TwoStageGSDwithVariousEndpoints(u0=0.08664+0.005,u1=0.08664,nStg1=123,
nStg2=123,alpha1=0.0026,beta1=1,alpha2=0.024,method="MINP",
w1squared=0.5,endpoint="survival",NId=0.005)

Note that the null hypothesis is $\mu_1 = 0.8664$ and $\mu_0 = \mu_1 + NId = 0.8664 + 0.005$. The simulation results are presented in Table 3.11.

Chapter 4

K-Stage Adaptive Confirmatory Design Methods

4.1 Test Statistics

For the same hypothesis test (3.1), the test statistic for the two-stage design can be generalized to any K-stage design:

$$
\begin{cases}
T_k = \sum_{i=1}^{k} p_i \text{ for MSP} \\
T_k = \prod_{i=1}^{k} p_i \text{ for MPP} \\
T_k = 1 - \Phi\left(\sum_{i=1}^{k} w_{ki} z_{1-p_i}\right) \text{ for MINP,}
\end{cases}
\tag{4.1}
$$

where p_i is the stagewise p-value at stage i and the subscript $k = 1, \ldots, K$. When the weight $w_{ki} = \sqrt{\frac{n_i}{\sum_{i=1}^{k} n_i}}$, T_k gives the test statistic for the classic group sequential design, where n_i is the same size of subsample from stage i.

The stopping rules at stage k are:

$$
\begin{cases}
\text{Stop for efficacy} & \text{if } T_k \leq \alpha_k, \\
\text{Stop for futility} & \text{if } T_k > \beta_k, \\
\text{Continue with adaptations if } \alpha_k < T_k \leq \beta_k,
\end{cases}
\tag{4.2}
$$

where $\alpha_k < \beta_k$ $(k = 1, \ldots, K-1)$, and $\alpha_K = \beta_K$. For convenience, α_k and β_k are called the efficacy and futility boundaries, respectively.

4.2 Determination of Stopping Boundary

We are going to present analytic, numerical, and simulation approaches to the K-stage design using nonparametric stopping boundaries and the error spending approach.

4.2.1   *Analytical Formulation for MSP*

The error-spending π_k in relation to the stopping boundaries for the first two stages is similar to (3.7) with α replaced by π_2, that is,

$$\begin{cases} \alpha_1 = \pi_1, \\ \alpha_2 = \sqrt{2\pi_2} + \alpha_1. \end{cases} \tag{4.3}$$

Chang (2010) provides analytical solutions for up to five-stage designs. For the third stage, we have

$$\pi_3 = \alpha_1\alpha_2\alpha_3 + \frac{1}{3}\alpha_2^3 + \frac{1}{6}\alpha_3^3 - \frac{1}{2}\alpha_1\alpha_2^2 - \frac{1}{2}\alpha_1\alpha_3^2 - \frac{1}{2}\alpha_2^2\alpha_3. \tag{4.4}$$

After we obtained α_1 and α_2, we can use (4.4) to obtain α_3 for the stopping boundary using numerical methods.

The general steps to determine the stopping boundaries for K-stage designs can be described as follows:

(1) Choose error spending $\pi_1, \ldots, \pi_{K-1}$, where $\sum_{k=1}^{K-1} \alpha_k < \alpha$.

(2) Calculate the error spending at the last stage: $\pi_K = \alpha - \sum_{k=1}^{K-1} \alpha_k$.

(3) Calculate the stopping boundary $\alpha_1, \alpha_2, \ldots, \alpha_K$, sequentially in that order.

Let's illustrate the steps with a three-stage design. Suppose the one-sided level of significance is $\alpha = 0.025$ and we want to spend less α at earlier stages and more on later stages. We choose $\pi_1 = 0.0025$ and $\pi_2 = 0.005$. Thus $\pi_3 = \alpha - \pi_1 - \pi_2 = 0.0175$. Furthermore, we can obtain from (3.7) the stopping boundary $\alpha_1 = \pi_1 = 0.0025$ and $\alpha_2 = \sqrt{2\pi_2} + \alpha_1 = 0.1025$. The stopping boundary α_3 can be solved numerically using software packages or by the trial-error method, which is $\alpha_1 = 0.49257$ (see the first column in Table 4.1).

Table 4.1: Stopping Boundaries of Three-Stage Design with MSP

π_1	0.00250	0.00500	0.00250	0.00500	0.00250	0.00500
π_2	0.00500	0.00500	0.00750	0.00750	0.01000	0.01000
π_3	0.01750	0.01500	0.01500	0.01250	0.01250	0.01000
α_1	0.00250	0.00500	0.00250	0.00500	0.00250	0.00500
α_2	0.10250	0.10500	0.12497	0.12747	0.14392	0.14642
α_3	0.49257	0.47226	0.47833	0.45580	0.46181	0.43628

Note: One-sided $\alpha = 0.025$, $\alpha_1 = \pi_1$, $\pi_3 = \alpha - \pi_1 - \pi_2$.

Table 4.2: Stopping Boundaries of Three-Stage Design with MPP

π_1	0.00250	0.00500	0.00250	0.00500	0.00250	0.00500
π_2	0.00500	0.00500	0.00750	0.00750	0.01000	0.01000
π_3	0.01750	0.01500	0.01500	0.01250	0.01250	0.01000
$\alpha_1(\times 10^{-3})$	2.50	5.00	2.50	5.00	2.50	5.00
$\alpha_2(\times 10^{-3})$	.83452	.94370	1.2518	1.4155	1.669	1.8874
$\alpha_3(\times 10^{-3})$	.71363	.65587	.67894	.60321	.61365	.52089

Note: One-sided $\alpha = 0.025, \alpha_1 = \pi_1, \pi_3 = \alpha - \pi_1 - \pi_2$.

4.2.2 Analytical Formulation for MPP

To determine the stopping boundaries for the first two stages with MPP, we use (3.9) but replace α by π_2:

$$\begin{cases} \alpha_1 = \pi_1, \\ \alpha_2 = \frac{\pi_2}{-\ln \alpha_1} \end{cases} \tag{4.5}$$

For the third stage, we have (Chang, 2015)

$$\alpha_3 = \frac{\pi_3}{\ln \alpha_2 \ln \alpha_1 - \frac{1}{2} \ln^2 \alpha_1}. \tag{4.6}$$

As soon as π_1, π_2, and π_3 are determined, α_1, α_2, and α_3 can be easily obtained from (4.5) and (4.6). Examples of stopping boundaries with MPP are presented in Table 4.2.

4.2.3 Stopping Boundaries for MINP

For MINP, the stopping boundaries can be determined through numerical integration or simulation (Table 4.3). Specifically, we use the two-stage adaptive design simulation R program with $\alpha_1 = \pi_1$. Run the simulation under H_0 using different values of α_2 until the power is equal to $\pi_1 + \pi_2$. After we obtain the stopping boundaries α_1 and α_2, we use the three-stage simulation R program with α_1 and α_2 that have been determined, but try different values of α_3 until the power is equal to $\alpha = 0.025$. Table 4.3 is the summary of the stopping boundary for equal information or equal weight ($w_1 = w_2 = \sqrt{2}$) designs. Note that (1) the efficacy stopping probability at stage i under H_0 is equal to π_i, which can be used to check the stopping boundaries α_i using simulations, and (2) the stopping boundaries in Table 4.1 through Table 4.3 are on p-scale, but one can convert them to z-scale by using the inverse-normal function: $z_{1-\alpha_i} = \Phi^{-1}(1 - \alpha_i)$.

For GSD with two to eight stages the O'Brien-Fleming stopping boundaries with equal information for the interim analyses and two-stage O'Brien-Fleming boundaries with various information times are presented in Appendix B.14.

Table 4.3: Stopping Boundaries of Three-Stage Design with MINP

π_1	0.00250	0.00500	0.00250	0.00500	0.00250	0.00500
π_2	0.00500	0.00500	0.00750	0.00750	0.01000	0.01000
π_3	0.01750	0.01500	0.01500	0.01250	0.01250	0.01000
α_1	0.00250	0.00500	0.00250	0.00500	0.00250	0.00500
α_2	0.00575	0.00653	0.00847	0.0091	0.0113	0.01182
α_3	0.02200	0.0198	0.0205	0.0184	0.0185	0.0164

Note: One-sided $\alpha = 0.025, \alpha_1 = \pi_1, \pi_3 = \alpha - \pi_1 - \pi_2$. 1 million runs.

4.3 Error-Spending Function

If we want the error-spending $\pi_1, \ldots, \pi_K$ to follow a certain trend (e.g., monotonic increase), we set up a so-called error-spending function $\pi^*(\tau_k)$, where τ_k is the information time or sample size fraction at the kth interim analysis. The commonly used error-spending functions (Figure 4.1) with one-sided α are the O'Brien-Fleming-like error-spending function

$$\pi^*(\tau_k) = 2\left\{1 - \Phi\left(\frac{z_{1-\alpha/2}}{\sqrt{\tau_k}}\right)\right\}, \tag{4.7}$$

the Pocock-like error-spending function

$$\pi^*(\tau_k) = \alpha \ln\left[1 + \frac{e-1}{\tau_k}\right], \tag{4.8}$$

and the power family

$$\pi^*(\tau_k) = \alpha\tau_k^\gamma, \tag{4.9}$$

where $\gamma > 0$ is a constant

The error-spending function $\pi^*(\tau_k)$ presents the cumulative error (α) spent up to the information time τ_k. Therefore, the error to spend at the kth stage with information time τ_k is determined by

$$\pi_k = \pi^*(\tau_k) - \pi^*(\tau_{k-1}). \tag{4.10}$$

After the error spending $\pi_1, \ldots, \pi_K$ are determined, the calculations of stopping boundaries $\alpha_1, \alpha_2, \ldots, \alpha_K$ can be carried out sequentially as illustrated previously. For instance, suppose we decide to use the power function $\pi^*(\tau_k) = \alpha\tau_k$ for the error-spending function and plan the interim analyses at the information time $\tau_1 = 1/3$ and $\tau_2 = 2/3$, and the final analysis at $\tau_3 = 1$. Substituting the τ_k into (4.9), we obtain $\pi^*(\tau_1 = 1/3) = \alpha/3$, $\pi^*(\tau_1 = 2/3) = \frac{2}{3}\alpha$, and $\pi^*(\tau_1 = 1) = \alpha$. In this case, $\pi_k = \frac{\alpha}{3}$. In other words, we spend α equally over the three analyses. The stopping

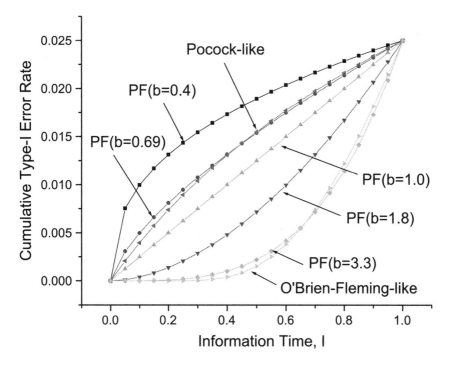

Figure 4.1: Error-Spending Functions

boundaries based on MSP and $\alpha = 0.025$ are: $\alpha_1 = 0.025/3$, $\alpha_2 = 0.137\,43$, and $\alpha_3 = 0.412\,24$.

4.4 Power and Sample Size

Let's illustrate the steps of using error-spending functions in GSDs. First, we need to select the number and timing of interim analyses based on the trial objectives.

(1) Determination of stopping boundary

If we don't want to choose the stopping boundaries in the tables provided in the book, we can determine the stopping boundaries α_i by running the simulations under H_0 using various different sets of stopping boundaries until the efficacy stopping probability (ESP[i] in the R function) match the errors spent π_i at each stage.

(2) Determination of the sample-size

After determining the stopping boundaries, keep everything the same, but change the treatment effect to the alternative hypothesis. Run the same simulation program using different sample sizes until the simulated power is close to the target power.

(3) Sensitivity analysis

Because the treatment difference and its variability are not exactly known, it is necessary to run the simulation under other critical conditions, which is referred to as sensitivity analysis or risk assessment.

Example 4.1 Three-Stage Adaptive Design

Again, we use the asthma trial discussed in Example 3.1. The estimated FEV1 improvement from baseline is 5% and 12% for the control and active groups, respectively, with a common standard deviation of $\sigma = 22\%$. We use an equal information design and the stopping boundaries from Table 4.3: $\alpha_1 = 0.0025$, $\alpha_2 = 0.00575$, $\alpha_3 = 0.022$ for efficacy boundaries, and $\beta_1 = \beta_2 = 0.5$ for the futility boundary. For 95% power with MINP at $\alpha = 0.025$ level, we use the following lines of code to invoke the simulation:

```
Nx = c(92,92,92); Ny = c(92,92,92); alphas = c(0.0025, 0.00575, 0.022); betas =
c(0.5, 0.5, 0.022)
TwoArmKStgGSDwithMINPNormalEndpoint(nSims=100000,    nStgs=3,    ux=0,
uy=0, NId=0, sigmax=0.22, sigmay=0.22)
TwoArmKStgGSDwithMINPNormalEndpoint(nSims=100000, nStgs=3, ux=0.05,
uy=0.12, NId=0, sigmax=0.22, sigmay=0.22)
TwoArmKStgGSDwithMINPNormalEndpoint(nSims=100000, nStgs=3, ux=0.05,
uy=0.10, NId=0, sigmax=0.22, sigmay=0.22)
```

(4) Operating characteristics

The operating characteristics obtained from the simulation are summarized in Table 4.4, where δ is the treatment difference.

The classical design requires 516 (86 per group for each stage) patients for 95% power. The sample size for the three-stage GSD requires average total sample size of 347, 368, and 440, respectively, for treatment effect $\delta = 0$, 0.07, and 0.05. We see the GSD can reduce expected sample size under H_0 and H_a. However, when the treatment effect $\delta = 0.05$, the sample size is larger and 445 patients will only provide 73.8% power, while classic design with 516 provides 73.3% power under this effect size. We will discuss how to improve the operating characteristic by means of sample size reestimation.

If we want to design this trial with MSP, we can use the following lines of code:

Table 4.4: Operating Characteristics with MINP

δ	ESP1	ESP2	ESP3	FSP1	FSP2	Power	$\bar{N}$
0	.0025	.0048	.0168	.5000	.1243	.024	347
0.07	.2500	.4500	.2400	.0156	.0004	.950	368
0.05	.1030	.2740	.3577	.0614	.0052	.735	440

Table 4.5: Operating Characteristics with MSP

δ	ESP1	ESP2	ESP3	FSP1	FSP2	Power	N̄
0	.003	.005	.017	.500	.369	.024	295
0.07	.259	.408	.264	.017	.025	.932	371
0.05	.101	.250	.353	.063	.114	.705	424

Nx = c(92,92,92); Ny = c(92,92,92); alphas = c(0.0025, 0.1025, 0.49257); betas = c(0.49257, 0.49257, 0.49257)
KStgGSDwithVariousEndpointsForMspMppMinp(ux=0, uy=0, sigmax=0.22, sigmay=0.22, nStgs=3, method="MSP", endpoint="normal", NId=0, nSims=100000)
    KStgGSDwithVariousEndpointsForMspMppMinp(ux=0.05, uy=0.12, sigmax=0.22, sigmay=0.22, nStgs=3, method="MSP", endpoint="normal", NId=0, nSims=100000)
    KStgGSDwithVariousEndpointsForMspMppMinp(ux=0.05, uy=0.10, sigmax=0.22, sigmay=0.22, nStgs=3, method="MSP", endpoint="normal", NId=0, nSims=100000)

The simulation results are presented in Table 4.5.

Example 4.2 Three-Stage ACS Adaptive Design

For the same ACS trial in Example 3.5, we now use three-stage design with MINP. The event rate of the primary endpoint is 14% for the control group and 12% for the test group. The total sample-size 1,152 will provide 90% power with the classical design. We choose $\alpha_1 = 0.005$, $\alpha_2 = 0.00653$, and $\alpha_3 = 0.0198$ from Table 4.3, and $\beta_1 = \beta_2 = 0.45$. The interim analyses will be performed at equal information intervals. We can try different sample sizes in the following code until it reaches the target power 85%.

Nx = c(1860,1860,1860); Ny = c(1860,1860,1860); alphas = c(0.005, 0.00653, 0.0198); betas = c(0.45, 0.45, 0.0198)
KStgGSDwithVariousEndpointsForMspMppMinp(ux=0, uy=0, nStgs=3, method="MINP", endpoint="binary", NId=0, nSims=10000)
KStgGSDwithVariousEndpointsForMspMppMinp(ux=0.12, uy=0.14, nStgs=3, method="MINP", endpoint="binary", NId=0, nSims=10000)

The operating characteristics are summarized in Table 4.6.
If one wants to use MPP instead of MINP, the following code can be invoked for the design simulation:

Table 4.6: Operating Characteristics with Three-Stage MINP

Case	ESP1	ESP2	ESP3	FSP1	FSP2	Power	Total N̄
Ho	.004	.005	.014	0.550	0.124	.024	6558
Ha	.218	.333	.297	0.047	0.003	.848	7941

Nx = c(1860,1860,1860); Ny = c(1860,1860,1860); alphas = c(0.0025, 0.00083452, 0.00071363); betas = c(1,1,0.00071363)
KStgGSDwithVariousEndpointsForMspMppMinp(ux=0,   uy=0,   nStgs=3, method="MPP", endpoint="binary", NId=0, nSims=100000)
KStgGSDwithVariousEndpointsForMspMppMinp(ux=0.12,   uy=0.14,   nStgs=3, method="MPP", endpoint="binary", NId=0, nSims=100000)

4.5 Error Spending Approach

It is good to know that when the prespecified error-spending function is followed, we can change the timing and number of the interim analyses without inflating the type-I error as long as such changes are not based on treatment difference. This is the advantage when we use an error-spending function and promise the function will be followed; such an extended GSD method is called error-spending approach.

Example 4.3 Changes in Number and Timing of Interim Analyses

An international, multicenter, randomized phase-III study to compare the test drug with a combination of drugs in patients with newly diagnosed multiple myeloma was designed using the O'Brien-Fleming spending function. The interim analysis was to be performed for 200 patients. The final analysis will be performed using 400 patients. The primary study objective is to assess the treatment difference in overall complete response rate (CR) obtained at the end of a 16-week induction phase. However, due to the complexity of the international trial, the data collection and validation became extremely challenging. It was decided that the investigator's assessment would be used because it is available much earlier than the assessment by the independent review committee (IRC) – the gold standard. However, the discrepancies between the two assessments are not known. The sponsor is concerned that if the trial is stopped based on the IDMC's recommendation, which is based on the investigator's assessment, it could be found later that the treatment difference is not significant based on the IRC's assessment. However, it is known that when the trial is stopped at the first interim analysis (IA), there will be more patients enrolled (about 300). Therefore, the sponsor decided to add a second interim analysis. With 300 patients (the exact number is based on the number of patients randomized at the first IA) at the second IA and based on the OB-F spending function (3.12), the error spent on the three analyses is $\pi_1 = 2\left[1 - \Phi\left(\frac{2.240}{\sqrt{200/400}}\right)\right] = 0.0016$, $\pi_2 = 2\left[1 - \Phi\left(\frac{2.240}{\sqrt{300/400}}\right)\right] - 0.0016 = 0.008$, and $\pi_3 = 2\left[1 - \Phi\left(2.240\right)\right] - 0.0096 = 0.015\,4$. The actual π_2 should be based on the actual number of patients at the second IA.

Chapter 5

Sample-Size Reestimation Design

5.1 Sample Size Reestimation Methods

Despite a great effort, we often face a high degree of uncertainty about parameters when designing a trial or justifying the sample-size at the design stage. This could involve the initial estimates of treatment effect and variability. When the uncertainty is greater, a classical design with a fixed sample-size is inappropriate. Instead, it is desirable to have a trial design that allows for reestimation of sample-size at the interim analysis. Several different methods have been proposed for sample-size reestimation (SSR), including the blinded, unblinded, and mixed methods.

5.1.1 *The Blinded Approach*

Wittes and Brittain (1990) and Gould and Shih (1992, 1998) discussed methods of blinded SSR. A blinded SSR assumes that the actually realized effect size estimate is not revealed through unblinding the treatment code. In blinded sample size reestimation, interim data are used to provide an updated estimate of a nuisance parameter without unblinding the treatment assignments. Nuisance parameters mentioned in this context are usually the variance for continuous outcomes. Wittes et al. (1999) and Zucker et al. (1999) investigated the performance of various blinded and unblinded SSR methods by simulation. They observed some slight type-I error violations in cases with small sample size. Friede and Kieser (2003, 2006) suggested a method of blinded sample size. Blinded sample reestimation is generally well accepted by regulators (ICH E-9, 1999). Proschan (2005) gives an excellent review on early research on two-stage SSR designs.

In clinical trials, the sample-size is determined by an estimated treatment difference and sample variability in the primary endpoint. Due to lack of knowledge of the test drug, the estimate of the variability is often not precise. As a result, the initially planned sample-size may turn out to be inappropriate and needs to be adjusted at interim analysis to ensure the power. A simple approach to dealing with nuisance parameter σ without unblinding the treatment code is to use the so-called *maximum information design*. The idea behind this approach is that recruitment continues until the prespecified information level is reached, i.e., $I = N/(2\hat{\sigma}^2) = I_{\max}$. For a given sample size, the information level reduces as the observed variance increases. The sample size per group for the two-group parallel design can be written in this familiar form:

$$N = \frac{2\sigma^2}{\delta^2}(z_{1-\alpha} + z_{1-\beta})^2, \tag{5.1}$$

where δ is treatment difference and σ is the common standard deviation.

For the normal endpoint, the treatment difference from the pooled (blinded) data follows a mixed normal distribution with the variance (Chang, 2014)

$$(\sigma^*)^2 = \sigma^2 + \left(\frac{\delta}{2}\right)^2, \tag{5.2}$$

where if we know (e.g., from a phase-II single arm trial) σ^2, we can estimate the treatment difference δ from (5.2). From (5.1) and (5.2), we can see that

$$N = 2\left(\frac{(\sigma^*)^2}{\delta^2} - \frac{1}{4}\right)(z_{1-\alpha} + z_{1-\beta})^2. \tag{5.3}$$

If we use the "lumped variance" $(\sigma^*)^2$ at the interim analysis in (5.3) from the blinded data, the new sample size required for the stage 2 is $N_2 = N - N_1$ or

$$N_2 = 2\left(\frac{(\hat{\sigma}^*)^2}{\delta} - \frac{1}{4}\right)(z_{1-\alpha} + z_{1-\beta})^2 - N_1, \tag{5.4}$$

where the interim sample size is N_1.

Formula (5.4) is the basis for the blinded sample-size reestimation.

5.1.2 *The Unblinded Approach*

In this method, we will not adjust the sample size if the observed treatment is zero or less. Otherwise, the sample size will be adjusted to meet the targeted conditional power but with the limit of the maximum sample size allowed due to the cost and time considerations:

$$n_2 = \min\left(N_{\max}, \frac{2\hat{\sigma}^2}{\hat{\delta}^2}\left[\frac{z_{1-\alpha} - w_1 z_{1-p_1}}{\sqrt{1-w_1^2}} - z_{1-cP}\right]^2\right), \quad \text{for } \hat{\delta} > 0, \tag{5.5}$$

where cP is the target conditional power, σ_0^2 is the common variance, n_2 is the sample-size per group at stage 2, and $z_x = \Phi^{-1}(x)$. Note that $\hat{\delta}$ and $\hat{\sigma}^2$ are MLEs from the unblinded data. A minimum sample size $N_{\min}$ can also be imposed.

Stopping Boundaries for SSR

The question is that when the sample size at the second stage change is based on p_1 from the first stage, will the stopping boundaries derived from the group sequential design in the previous chapter still be valid?

For MINP, $T_2 = \sqrt{\tau_1}z_1 + \sqrt{1-\tau_1}z_2$, where the information time $\tau_1 = n_1/N$, under H_0, z_1 and z_2 are iid from $N(0,1)$, which seems to imply that sample size modification will not affect the stopping boundaries because a linear combination of normal variables is a normal distribution. However, since τ_1 is a function of sample size and sample size adjustment is dependent on z_1 or p_1, T_2 is no longer a linear combination of two independent standard normal distributions. As a result, the stopping boundaries from a GSD have to be changed in order to control the type-I error.

For MSP and MPP, the conditional distribution of p_2 given be p_1 must be uniformly distributed in [0,1] or p-clud under the null hypothesis H_0. We can easily to check this condition. If $p_2 = 1 - \Phi\left(\bar{X}_2\sqrt{\frac{n_2}{\sigma}}\right)$, where the second stage mean $\bar{X}_2$ is independent of p_1 but the sample size at the second stage n_2 is a function of p_1. Therefore, p_1 and p_2 are independent and uniformly distributed in [0,1] for the sequential design without sample-size reestimation, but they are not independent anymore when the sample n_2 is adjusted based on p_1 directly or indirectly and we cannot guarantee the two p-values are p-clud. Fortunately, when the null hypothesis is true and regardless of sample size n_2, p_2 is uniformly distributed in [0,1] or p-clud. This is because $\bar{X}_2\sqrt{\frac{n_2}{\sigma}}$ has the standard normal distribution regardless of the sample size n_2 as long as H_0 is true. As a result, the stopping boundaries discussed in previous chapters can be used for MSP and MPP. For MINP, the weights w_{ki} must be fixed; otherwise, the same stopping boundary for GSD cannot be used for SSR design.

Comparison of Conditional Power

For adaptive designs, conditional power is often a better measure than power regarding the efficiency. The differences in conditional power between different methods are dependent on the stagewise p-value from the first stage. From Table 5.1 and Figure 5.1, it can be seen that conditional power for MSP is uniformly higher for p_1 around 0.1 than the other two methods. Therefore, if you believe that p_1 will be somewhere between (0.005, 0.18), then MSP is much more efficient than MPP and MINP; otherwise, MPP and MINP are better.

Table 5.1: Conditional Powers as Function of p-Value at Stage 1

Method	0.010	0.050	0.100	p_1 0.150	0.180	0.220
				Power		
MSP	0.880	0.847	0.788	0.685	0.572	0.044
MPP	0.954	0.712	0.567	0.516	0.485	0.453
MINP	0.937	0.802	0.686	0.595	0.547	0.490

Note: $\alpha_1 = 0.0025$. $N_2 = 200$, effect size $= 0.2$, no futility binding.

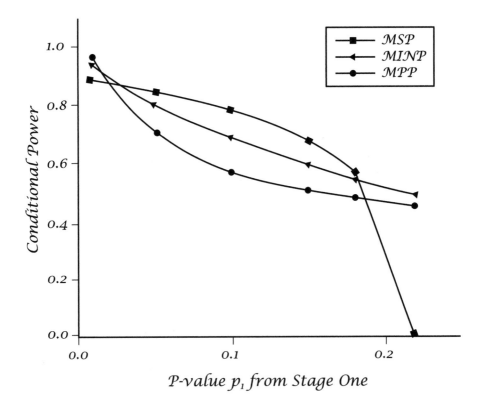

Figure 5.1:   Conditional Power versus p-Value from Stage 1

Example 5.1: Unblinded Sample-Size Reestimation Trial

Assume the standardized effect size is 0.33 in a two-group adaptive design with SSR. Let's use $\alpha_1 = 0.005$, $\beta_1 = 0.205$, $\alpha_2 = 0.205$, 0.0038, and 0.0226 for MSP, MPP, and MINP, respectively. Note that when $p_1 > \beta_1 = 0.205$, there is no possibility of rejecting the null hypothesis at the second stage for MSP. The sample size for the first stage is $N_1 = 80$ and the minimum and maximum sample-sizes are $N_{\min} = 160$ and $N_{\max} = 320$ per group. Table

Table 5.2: Comparisons of Adaptive Methods

Method	α_2	$\bar{\mathrm{N}}$o	$\bar{\mathrm{N}}$a	Power (H_a)	N_s	Power (H_s)
MSP	.2050	121	170	86%	179	75%
MPP	.0038	123	179	87%	189	76%
MINP	.0226	122	173	87%	183	77%

Note: $\alpha_1 = 0.005$, $\beta_1 = 0.205$, H_a: $\delta = 0.33$, H_s:$\delta = 0.28$.

5.2 gives a quick comparison of different methods, where $\bar{\mathrm{N}}$o is the expected sample-size under the null hypothesis, $\bar{\mathrm{N}}$a is the expected sample-size under the alternative hypothesis, and $\bar{\mathrm{N}}$s is the expected sample-size under the condition when there is a smaller effect size than that in H_a. All designs have a 90% target conditional power. Overall, MIMP and MPP designs perform very similarly, while MSP slightly underperformed.

```
# Example 5.1
# Checking Type-I error with MINP ##
                                    powerTwoStageUnblindSSRnormal-
Endpoint(u0=0,u1=0,sigma=1, nStg1=80, nStg2=80, alpha1=0.0026, beta1=0.205,
alpha2=0.024, cPower=0.9, method="MINP", nMax=320, w1=0.7071)
## Power with MINP under Ha
                                    powerTwoStageUnblindSSRnormalEnd-
point(u0=0,u1=0.33,sigma=1, nStg1=80, nStg2=80, alpha1=0.0026, beta1=0.205,
alpha2=0.024, cPower=0.9, method="MINP", nMax=320, w1=0.7071)
## Power with MINP Under Hs
                                    powerTwoStageUnblindSSRnormalEnd-
point(u0=0,u1=0.28,sigma=1, nStg1=80, nStg2=80, alpha1=0.0026, beta1=0.205,
alpha2=0.024, cPower=0.9, method="MINP", nMax=320, w1=0.7071)
# Checking Type-I error with MSP ##
              powerTwoStageUnblindSSRnormalEndpoint(u0=0,u1=0,sigma=1,
nStg1=80, nStg2=80, alpha1=0.0026, beta1=0.205, alpha2=0.21463, cPower=0.9,
method="MSP", nMax=320)
## Power with MSP under Ha
              powerTwoStageUnblindSSRnormalEndpoint(u0=0,u1=0.33,sigma=1,
nStg1=80, nStg2=80, alpha1=0.0026, beta1=0.205, alpha2=0.21463, cPower=0.9,
method="MSP", nMax=320)
## Power with MSP under Hs
              powerTwoStageUnblindSSRnormalEndpoint(u0=0,u1=0.28,sigma=1,
nStg1=80, nStg2=80, alpha1=0.0026, beta1=0.205, alpha2=0.21463, cPower=0.9,
method="MSP", nMax=320)
## Checking Type-I error with MPP##
                                    powerTwoStageUnblindSSRnormal-
```

Endpoint(u0=0,u1=0,sigma=1, nStg1=80, nStg2=80, alpha1=0.0025, beta1=0.205, alpha2=0.0038, cPower=0.9, method="MPP",nMax=320)

Power with MPP##

powerTwoStageUnblindSSRnormalEndpoint(u0=0,u1=0.33,sigma=1,nStg1=80, nStg2=80, alpha1=0.0025, beta1=0.205, alpha2=0.0038, cPower=0.9, method="MPP",nMax=320)

Power with MPP##

powerTwoStageUnblindSSRnormalEndpoint(u0=0,u1=0.28,sigma=1,nStg1=80, nStg2=80, alpha1=0.0025, beta1=0.205, alpha2=0.0038, cPower=0.9, method="MPP",nMax=320)

The simulation program for the two-stage SSR design with various endpoints is provided in the Appendix.

5.1.3 *The Mixed Approach*

In this method, the sample-size adjustment has the similar formulation as for unblinded SSR (5.5) but replaces the term $\frac{\hat{\sigma}^2}{\hat{\delta}^2}$ with blinded estimate $\frac{\hat{\sigma}^*}{\delta_0}$:

$$n_2 = \min\left(N_{\max}, 2\left(\frac{\hat{\sigma}^*}{\delta_0}\right)^2\left[\frac{z_{1-\alpha} - w_1 z_{1-p_1}}{\sqrt{1-w_1^2}} - z_{1-cP}\right]^2\right), \quad \hat{\delta} > 0, \quad (5.6)$$

where δ_0 is the initial estimation of treatment difference and $(\hat{\sigma}^*)^2$ is the variance estimated from the blinded data:

$$(\hat{\sigma}^*)^2 = \frac{\sum_{i=1}^{N}(x_i - \bar{x})^2}{N}.$$

To reduce the sample size when the drug is ineffective (δ is very small or negative), when we use (5.6), we need to have the futility boundary. Since the sample size adjustment is based on the blinded value $\frac{\hat{\sigma}^*}{\delta_0}$, while z_{1-p_1} and the futility boundary are based on unblinded data, we call this method the mixed method.

Like the blinded maximum information SSR, the sample size adjustment with the mixed method will not release the treatment difference to the public. Most importantly the SSR method is much more efficient than all other methods: when the true treatment is lower than the initial estimation, the sample size will increase automatically to effectively prevent a large drop in power. However, the problem with this method is that it will increase the sample size dramatically even when the treatment effect is zero. Therefore, to avoid that, we have to use a futility boundary; for example, when the observed treatment effect is zero or less, the trial will be stopped.

Table 5.3: Comparisons of SSR Mixed Methods

	$\delta = 0$		$\delta = 0.25$		$\delta = 0.3$				$\delta = 0.35$	
	$\sigma = 3$		$\sigma = 3$		$\sigma = 3$		$\sigma = 4$		$\sigma = 3$	
	$\bar{N}$	Err	$\bar{N}$	Pow	$\bar{N}$	Pow	$\bar{N}$	Pow	$\bar{N}$	Pow
Classical	2100	.025	2100	.77	2100	.90	2100	.68	2100	.966
MaxInfo	1800	.024	2100	.77	2100	.90	2686	.78	2100	.966
Unblind SSR	2264	.025	2233	.82	2098	.92	2277	.74	1932	.972
Mixed SSR	1992	.028	2189	.83	2071	.93	2827	.84	1971	.974

Note: $\alpha = 0.025$, cPower=90%.

5.2 Comparisons of SSR Methods

To reduce the sample size under H_0, we use futility boundary $\beta_1 = 0.5$. In other words, if the one-sided p-value at the interim analysis is larger than 0.5, the trial will stop due to futility. There is no early efficacy stopping in the comparisons. For MaxInfo and Mixed SSR designs, we choose $N_{max} = 4000$/group, $N_{min} = 1800$/group, and $N_1 = 900$/group and for unblind SSR design, $N_{max} = 3000$/group, $N_{min} = 1600$/group, and $N_1 = 800$/group so that all designs have approximately the same expected sample size of 2,100 under scenario $\sigma = 3$ and $\delta = 0.3$.

The simulation results (Table 5.3) show that the mixed SSR performs well in all conditions – better than the unblind SSR. The unblind SSR design fails to protect the power when σ is underestimated and the unblind SSR design requires a larger sample size of 2,264 per group versus 1,992 per group for the mixed SSR design. The MaxInfo design can somewhat protect power comparing the classic design when variance is underestimated (74% versus 68%), but it cannot protect the power at all when the treatment effect is overestimated (power =77%, the same as for the classic design). However, simulation results show there are slightly type-I error inflations with the mixed SSR design; therefore, we can adjust the rejection criterion to $p < 0.022$ (instead of $p < 0.025$) for mixed methods. With this adjustment, the mixed method will strongly control the type-I error and still perform very well.

For the mixed SSR method, the maximum sample size N_{max} should be about $2N$, where N_{min} should be about the same as the initial sample size N for the classic design. Increasing N_{max} more than $2N$ will not be effective in increasing the power.

Example 5.2 Myocardial Infarction Prevention Trial

This example is based on the case presented by Cui, Hung, and Wang (1999). In a phase-III, two-arm trial to evaluate the effect of a new drug on the prevention of myocardial infarction in patients undergoing coronary artery bypass graft surgery, a sample-size of 300 patients per group will provide 95%

Table 5.4: Comparison of Classical and Adaptive Designs

Design	\bar{N}	Power (%)	\bar{N}	Power (%)	\bar{N}	Power (%)	\bar{N}_0
	\multicolumn{7}{c}{Event Rate in the Test Group P_T}						
	0.10		0.11		0.14		0.22
Classical	290	98	290	95	290	72	290
GSD	220	98	236	95	270	72	224
SSR	236	98	260	96	310	78	238

Note: $\alpha_1 = 0.026$, $\beta_1 = 0.5$, $N_{\max} = 410$/group, target cP $= 0.95$.

power to detect a 50% reduction in incidence from 22% to 11% at the one-sided significance level $\alpha = 0.025$. Although the sponsor is confident about the incidence of 22% in the control group, the sponsor is not that sure about the 11% incidence rate in the test group. For this reason we perform the simulations to compare the classic, two-stage GSD and two-stage SSR designs under three different event rates for the test group: 0.10, 0.11, and 0.14. The O'Brien-Fleming efficacy stopping boundary is used and $\beta_1 = 0.5$ is used for the futility stopping. For the GSD, interim analysis is performed based on sample size 150/group and the maximum sample size is 300 per group. For SSR design, the interim analysis will be performed at sample size $= 100$ patients. The minimum sample size is 200/group and the maximum sample size is 410/group if the trial is continued to the stage 2.

The simulation results are presented in Table 5.4. From the simulation results, there are several noticeable features of adaptive designs: the unblind and mixed SSR methods give almost identical results for the binary endpoint, so we just present one set of results. The SSR design provides some level of power protection when the treatment is lower than expected, but GSD fails to protect power in this case. For the classical design, if we increase the sample size to 410/group, then the sample size will increase for all the scenarios, which we don't want. We want to increase the sample size substantially only when the treatment effect is lower.

5.3 K-Stage Sample Size Reestimation Trial

For K-stage design with MINP, the conditional power at stage k can be expressed as (Jennison and Turnbull, 2000):

$$cP_\delta = \Phi \left(\frac{Z_k \sqrt{I_k} - z_{1-\alpha} \sqrt{I_K} + (I_K - I_k)\delta}{\sqrt{I_K - I_k}} \right), \quad k = 1, \ldots, K - 1, \qquad (5.7)$$

where information level

$$I_k = \left(\frac{\sigma_A^2}{n_{Ak}} + \frac{\sigma_B^2}{n_{Bk}} \right)^{-1}.$$

Here n_{Ak} and n_{Bk} are subsample sizes in treatment groups A and B.

The Bayesian predictive power at stage k is given by

$$P_\delta = \Phi\left(\frac{Z_k\sqrt{I_k} - z_{1-\alpha}\sqrt{I_K}}{\sqrt{I_K - I_k}}\right), \, k = 1, \ldots, K - 1. \tag{5.8}$$

However, caution should be taken when using (5.7) and (5.8) since conditional power and predictive power should be generally dependent on the error-spending function or stopping boundary we have chosen, but (5.7) and (5.8) are free of the error-spending function. The sample size required can be solved numerical when the conditional power or predictive power is given.

5.4 Summary

(1) Futility stopping can reduce the sample-size when the null is true. The futility boundary is suggested because in the case of a very small effect size, to continue the trial will require an unrealistically large sample-size, and an increased sample-size to N_{max} still may not have enough power.

(2) From the α-control point of view, for the methods in this chapter (MSP, MPP, and MINP with unblind SSR or mixed SSR), the algorithm for sample-size adjustment does not have to be predetermined; instead, it can be determined after we observed the results from the interim analysis.

(3) It might be a concern if the sample-size is based on a predetermined algorithm, because IDMC's determination of the new sample-size will actually require the disclosure of the efficacy information for the trial. There is a simple way to handle it: the use of the mixed SSR method.

(4) Power is an estimation, made at the initial design stage, of the probability of rejecting the null hypothesis. Therefore, it is less important when the sample-size can be adjusted at IA. In other words, the initial total sample-size is irrelevant to the final sample-size (it is only relevant for budgeting and operational planning), but the sample-size at the first stage is relevant; N_{mim} and N_{max} are relevant to the power.

(5) For adaptive designs, the conditional power is more important than the power. MSP often is superior over other methods in terms of conditional power. The nonbinding futility rule is currently adopted by regulatory bodies. With nonbinding futility boundaries, MSP is often superior over other methods.

(6) Through simulations, we conclude that the mixed method is a very effective tool for SSR design, better than other blind and unblind SSR methods. We highly recommend the mixed approach in practice. As to the slight inflation of type-I error with the mixed method (not related to the unblinding at all), we can use a smaller α from simulations to control the type-I error.

Chapter 6

Special Two-Stage Group Sequential Trials

6.1 Event-Based Design

The methods discussed for survival analyses so far are based on the number of patients at each stage, instead of number of events. The reason for this is that the methods are based on the assumption of independent stagewise statistics. Therefore, the first N_1 patients enrolled will be used for the first interim analysis regardless of whether they have the event or not. Strictly speaking, for the commonly used log-rank test statistics based on number of events, the test statistics at different stages,

$$T\left(\hat{D}_k\right) = \sqrt{\frac{\hat{D}_k}{2}} \ln \frac{\hat{\lambda}_1}{\hat{\lambda}_2} \sim N\left(\sqrt{\frac{D_k}{2}} \ln \frac{\lambda_1}{\lambda_2}, 1\right), \qquad (6.1)$$

are not independent, where D_k is the number of events at the kth stage. However, Breslow and Haug (1977) and Canner (1997) showed that the independent normal approximation works well for small D_k. The relationship between the number of deaths and number of patients is simple under exponential survival models. Whether based on the number of events or patients, the results are very similar (Chang, 2007c, and 2014, Chapter 4). Other methods for adaptive design with a survival endpoint can be found from work by Li, Shih, and Wang (2005), and Jenkins, Stone, and Jennison (2011). Practically, the accrual has to continue in most cases when collecting the data and performing the interim analysis; it is often the case that at the time when interim analysis is done, most or all patients are enrolled. What is the point to have the interim analysis? The answer is that a positive interim analysis would allow the drug to be on the market earlier.

6.2 Equivalence Trial

We now discuss the two-stage adaptive design that allows for sample-size adjustment based on information at the first stage. The hypothesis for the equivalence study is defined by (2.5). The key for the adaptive equivalence trial is to define an appropriate stagewise p-value; we can use a p-value based on a subsample from the kth stage, i.e.,

$$p_k = 1 - \Phi\left(T_k\right), \qquad (6.2)$$

where

$$T_k = \frac{\delta_{NI} - |\bar{x}_{kR} - \bar{x}_{kT}|}{\hat{\sigma}_k\sqrt{\frac{2}{n_k}}}. \qquad (6.3)$$

Note that $\delta - |\bar{x}_{kR} - \bar{x}_{kT}|$ has a folded normal distribution with mean $\mu = \delta_{NI} - |\mu_R - \mu_T|$ and variance $\text{var}(|\bar{x}_{kR} - \bar{x}_{kT}|) < \hat{\sigma}_k\sqrt{\frac{2}{n_k}}$ (Tsagris, Beneki, and Hassani, 2014).

Example 6.1 Adaptive Equivalence LDL Trial

Suppose in designing an equivalence trial, the equivalence margin is assumed to be $\delta = 0.2$ and the standard deviation is $\sigma = 0.72$. The group sequential equivalence trial is designed with the two-sided $\alpha = 0.05$. An interim analysis is planned and the stagewise sample size is $n_1 = n_2 = 200$ per group.

To study the operating characteristics, we use the following R code to invoke the simulation:

```
## Example 6.1: Type I error control with O'Brien-Fleming Boundary is conservative since the pdf of the test statistics has heavy tails.
                                        TwoStageEquivGSDwithNormal-
Endpoint(du=0.2, sigma=0.72, Eqd=0.2, nStg1=200, nStg2=200, alpha1=0.0052,
beta1=1, alpha2=0.048, w1squared=0.5, nSims=1000000)
## Example 6.1: Power GSD for Equivalence Trial
    TwoStageEquivGSDwithNormalEndpoint(du=0,    sigma=0.72,    Eqd=0.2,
nStg1=200, nStg2=200, alpha1=0.0052, beta1=1, alpha2=0.048, w1squared=0.5,
nSims=100000)
## Example 6.1: Type I error control
                                        TwoStageEquivGSDwithNormal-
Endpoint(du=0.2, sigma=0.72, Eqd=0.2, nStg1=200, nStg2=200, alpha1=0.0055,
beta1=1, alpha2=0.024, w1squared=0.5, nSims=1000000)
## Example 6.1: Power GSD for Equivalence Trial
    TwoStageEquivGSDwithNormalEndpoint(du=0,    sigma=0.72,    Eqd=0.2,
nStg1=200, nStg2=200, alpha1=0.0055, beta1=1, alpha2=0.024, w1squared=0.5,
nSims=100000)
```

If we treat T_k in (6.3) as normal distribution and the standard normal distribution under the null hypothesis and apply the common O'Brien-Fleming boundary ($\alpha_1 = 0.0052$ and $\alpha_2 = 0.048$), the type-error rate will be around 4.8%. This is because we did not use the variance $\text{var}(|\bar{x}_{kR} - \bar{x}_{kT}|)$ but a larger one $\hat{\sigma}_k \sqrt{\frac{2}{n_k}}$ and T_k follows a folded normal distribution. The simulation results show that the expected sample size is about $N = 399$ and 365 per group under H_0 and H_a, respectively, for a design with 95% power. If we adjust the stopping boundary to $\alpha_1 = 0.0085$ and $\alpha_2 = 0.048$ so that the type-one error will be 5%, the sample-size under the null condition with treatment difference equals the equivalence margin 0.2, the expected sample-size is $\bar{N} = 398/\text{group}$; under the alternative condition with no treatment difference, the expected sample size is $\bar{N} = 339/\text{group}$ for 95% power.

6.3 Adaptive Design with Farrington-Manning Margin

There are two ways to define the noninferiority margin: (1) a prefixed noninferiority (NI) margin and (2) a noninferiority margin proportional to the effect of the active control group, i.e., Farrington-Manning noninferiority margin. The former has been discussed in Chapter 2. We now discuss the latter. The Farrington-Manning noninferiority test was proposed for a classical design with a binary endpoint (Farrington and Manning, 1990), but can be extended to adaptive designs with different endpoints. The null hypothesis can be defined as $H_0 : u_t - (1 - \delta_{NI}) u_c \leq 0$, where $0 < \delta_{NI} < 1$, u_t and u_c are the responses (mean, proportion, median survival time) for test and control groups, respectively. The test statistic is defined as

$$z_k = \frac{\hat{u}_t - (1 - \delta_{NI}) \hat{u}_c}{\sqrt{\sigma_t^2/n_k + (1 - \delta_{NI})\sigma_c^2/n_k}}, \tag{6.4}$$

where $\sigma_t^2 = var(\hat{u}_t)$ and $\sigma_c^2 = var(\hat{u}_c)$ are given by Table 2.1, and can be calculated based on data from stage k (not cumulative data):

$$T_k = 1 - \Phi(z_k), \tag{6.5}$$

It is important to know that there is a variance reduction in comparison with the prefixed NI margin approach, in which the variance is $\sigma_t^2 + \sigma_c^2$ instead of $\sigma_t^2 + (1 - \delta_{NI})^2\sigma_c^2$. Therefore, the Farrington-Manning test is usually much more powerful than the fixed margin approach.

Example 6.2: Adaptive Design with Farrington-Manning NI Margin

Suppose in designing a cholesterol trial, the treatment effect in reducing LDL is estimated to 20% with a standard deviation of 14%. Suppose we design a noninferiority trial using an NI margin for the Farrington-Manning test with $\delta_{NI} = 0.1$. The sample-size 300 per group will provide 90% power for the NI test at a level of significance $\alpha = 0.025$. The interim analysis will be conducted on 50% patients with an O'Brien-Fleming boundary. The simulation program

(R function) is presented in the appendix and the following R code can be used to invoke the R function for power and sample size calculation.

powerTwoStageFarringtonManningNIwithSSRnormalEndpoint(u0=0.20,u1=0.20, sigma=0.08, nStg1=150, nStg2=150, alpha1=0.0026, beta1=0.205, alpha2=0.024, NId=0.1, cPower=0.9, method="MINP", nMax=320, w1=0.7071)

6.4 Noninferiority Trial with Paired Binary Data

6.4.1 *Noninferiority Hypothesis*

Most commonly used noninferiority trials are based on parallel, two-group designs, which we have discussed in Chapter 3. In this section, we study how to design an adaptive noninferiority trial with paired binary data.

Noninferiority of a diagnostic test to the standard is a common issue in medical research. For instance, we may be interested in determining if a new diagnostic test is noninferior to the standard reference test because the new test might be inexpensive to the extent that some small inferior margin in sensitivity or specificity may be acceptable. Noninferiority trials are also found to be useful in clinical trials, such as image studies, where the data are collected in pairs. In such a trial sensitivity and specificity are often the two coprimary endpoints. It is usually required to demonstrate that the method is superior to the control in sensitivity and noninferior in specificity.

Let Y_1 and Y_2 be, respectively, binary response variables of treatments 1 and 2 with the joint distribution $P(Y_1 = i; Y_2 = j) = p_{ij}$ for $i = 0, 1; j = 0, 1$. $\sum_{i=0}^{1} \sum_{j=0}^{1} p_{ij} = 1$. Paired data are commonly displayed in a 2×2 contingency table (Table 6.1).

Nam (1997) proposed the following asymptotic test for paired data:

$$H_0 : p_{10} - p_{01} - \delta_{NI} \leq 0 \text{ vs. } H_a: H_0, \tag{6.6}$$

where $\delta_{NI} < 0$ is the noninferiority margin. Nam (1997) proved that the test statistic, defined as

$$Z = \frac{\hat{\varepsilon}\sqrt{n}}{\hat{\sigma}}, \tag{6.7}$$

Table 6.1: Matched-Pair Data

	Test		Total
Control	1	0	
1	x_{11}	x_{10}	
0	x_{01}	x_{00}	
Total			n

follows approximately the normal distribution for large n,

$$Z \sim N\left(\frac{\sqrt{n}\varepsilon}{\sigma}, 1\right),$$

(6.8)

where

$$\begin{cases} \hat{\varepsilon} = \hat{p}_{10} - \hat{p}_{01} - \delta_{NI}, \\ \hat{p}_{ij} = x_{ij}/n, \\ \hat{\sigma}^2 = 2\tilde{p}_{01} + \delta_{NI} - \delta_{NI}^2, \end{cases}$$

(6.9)

and $\tilde{p}_{10}$ is the restricted MLE of p_{10},

$$\begin{cases} \tilde{p}_{01} = \frac{-b+\sqrt{b^2-8c}}{4}, \\ b = (2 + \hat{p}_{01} - \hat{p}_{10})\delta_{NI} - \hat{p}_{01} - \hat{p}_{10}, \\ c = -\hat{p}_{01}\delta_{NI}(1 - \delta_{NI}). \end{cases}$$

(6.10)

Here $\varepsilon = E(\hat{\varepsilon})$ and $\sigma = E(\hat{\sigma})$ can be obtained by replacing $\hat{p}_{ij}$ with p_{ij} $(i = 0, 1; j = 0, 1)$ in the corresponding expression (6.7).

Comparing (6.9) with (2.1), we can view $\hat{\sigma}^2/2$ in (6.9) as the equivalent variance for two-group normal endpoint adaptive design. All the programming algorithms will be the same. This approach of equivalent variance will be used frequently in the rest of the book.

6.4.2 *Prostate Cancer Diagnostic Trial*

Preliminary Data for Trial Design

The adaptive design considerations will be oriented toward comparisons of the diagnostic performance of two scanning methods separately for sensitivity (using data from true positive patients) and specificity (using data from true negative patients).

The two methods (Method 1 is a good standard) for the detection of metastatic disease in a group of subjects with known prostate cancer use standardized clinical endpoints of documented disease including clinical outcome, serial PSA levels, contrast enhanced CT scans and radionuclide bone scans. A small study was conducted on a group of matched patients. The sensitivity and specificity are presented in Table 6.2.

Table 6.2: Sensitivity and Specificity

Method	Sensitivity	Specificity
1	63%	80%
2	84%	80%

Table 6.3: Positive Patients per CT/Bone Scan

Method 2	Method 1 Positive	Method 1 Negative
Positive	62%	20%
Negative	3%	15%

Table 6.4: Negative Patients per CT/Bone Scan

Method 2	Method 1 Negative	Method 1 Positive
Negative	60%	10%
Positive	10%	20%

The 2×2 table of the data for the McNemar's test in positive patients per CT/bone scan is given in Table 6.3. The 2×2 table of the data for the McNemar's test in negative patients per CT/bone scan is given in Table 6.4.

The Effectiveness Requirements

The requirements for gaining the regulatory approval are defined as follows:

- Superiority on sensitivity with 10% margin (point estimate) and NI on specificity with 7.5% margin (CI); the hypothesis testing is based on the results from 2 out of 3 image readers.
- Statistical methods: McNemar's test with and without cluster adjustment. However, since we don't have data about the cluster, our sample size calculation will be based on testing without considering clustering.

The effectiveness claim will be based primarily on subject level results, that is, a diagnosis of whether or not the patient has any evidence of metastatic prostate cancer, disregarding the number of sites of disease. The analyses of lesions will provide additional information on the ability of the diagnostic tests to determine localization and staging of the disease. For this reason, the sample size will be based on analysis results on the subject level. It is required that Method 2 have at least a 10% improvement (based on a point estimate) over Method 1 in sensitivity and be noninferior to Method 1 in specificity with a margin of 7.5%.

Design for Sensitivity

For the purpose of comparison, we first calculate the sample size required for the classical design. Given the data in Table 6.3, i.e., $p_{10} = 0.2$ and $p_{01} = 0.03$, for a 95% power at a level of significance 2.5% (one-sided), 82 pairs are required based on McNemar's test.

Table 6.5: Operating Characteristics of AD under Ha for Sensitivity

	α_1	α_2	ESP	Power	$\bar{N}_a$	FSP	$\bar{N}_o$	N_{max}
OF	.00260	.02400	.263	.95	73.0	0.45	65.3	84
PF	.00625	.02173	.429	.95	67.5	0.45	66.7	86
Pocock	.01470	.01470	.625	.95	63.2	0.45	71.0	92

Note: $\beta_1 = 0.5$, the proportions of shifting: $p_{10} = 0.2$, $p_{01} = 0.03$.

For group sequential designs (GSDs), three different error-spending functions are considered: (1) the O'Brien-Fleming-like error-spending function (OF), (2) the power-function with $\rho = 2$ (PF), and (3) the Pocock-like error-spending function (Pocock).

Given the data in Table 6.4 and a 95% power, we design the group sequential trial with one interim analysis at 50% information time. The simulation results are presented in Table 6.5. To choose an "optimal" design, we perform the following comparisons (Table 6.5):

(1) Comparing the results from the OF and the PF designs, we can see that the latter requires a smaller expected sample size ($\bar{N}_a$), a 7.5% reduction (73 versus 67.5 pairs) because the PF design has a larger early efficacy stopping probability (ESP = 0.429) than the OF design (ESP = 0.263). The maximum sample size is almost the same for the two designs. Therefore, the PF design with $\rho = 2$ is a better design than the OF design.

(2) Comparing the results from the Pocock and PF designs, we can see that the latter require a smaller maximum sample-size (86 versus 92), a smaller expected sample-size under H_0 (66.7 versus 71.0), and a larger expected sample size under H_a (67.5 versus 63.2). We further compare the sample sizes required under other conditions, such as H_0.

(3) Under H_0: $p_{10} = p_{01} = 0.2$, the expected sample sizes are 65.3, 66.7, and 71 pairs for the OF, the PF, and the Pocock designs, respectively. The expected sample sizes under H_0 are thus similar for the OF and PF designs while being smaller than that for the Pocock design. The early futility stopping probabilities (EFP) are almost identical, i.e., 45% for all three designs, which deviates from the theoretical value 50% due to approximation in normality. Based on these comparisons, we believe the design with PF ($\rho = 2$) is the best design among the three (Table 6.5). The design can save about 18% in the expected sample size from the classical design (67 versus 82 pairs).

Design for Specificity

Like the GSD for sensitivity, we start with a classical design for specificity. Given the data in Table 6.4, i.e., $p_{10} = 0.1$ and $p_{01} = 0.1$, the calculation indicates that 322 pairs are required for an 85% power at a level of significance

Table 6.6: Operating Characteristics of Adaptive Design for Specificity

	α_1	α_2	N_{max}	ESP	Power	$\bar{N}_a$	FSP	$\bar{N}_o$
OF	.00260	.02400	500	.206	.942	354	0.47	335
PF	.00625	.02173	500	.328	.940	336	0.47	335
Pocock	.01470	.01470	500	.454	.931	324	0.47	335

of 2.5% (one-sided) based on Nam's test (1997) and the sample size calculation method presented earlier (Table 6.5).

We use the same three error-spending functions for the adaptive trial for specificity: (1) OF, (2) PF with $\rho = 2$, and (3) the Pocock. All designs have two stages and the interim analysis will be performed at 50% information time with a sample size of 161 pairs. The sample size adjustment is based on a targeted conditional power of 90% and the maximum sample size N_{max} is 500 pairs. In all designs we use the futility boundary $\beta_1 = 0.5$, which means approximately that if at interim analysis we observe $\hat{p}_{10} - \hat{p}_{01} - \delta_{NI} \leq 0$, we will stop the trial for futility.

The simulation results are presented in Table 6.6, where EEP and $\bar{N}_a$ are the early efficacy stopping probability and expected sample size when H_a ($p_{10} = p_{01} = 0.1$) is true, respectively.

Following the same steps for comparing different adaptive designs in sensitivity, we find the PF design is better than the OF design. To evaluate the PF design against the Pocock design, we need to perform the simulations under $H_0 : p_{10} - p_{01} - \delta_{NI} = 0$ ($p_{10} = 0.1$, $p_{01} = 0.175$, and $\delta_{NI} = 0.075$). Under this null hypothesis, the OF, PF, and Pocock designs have almost the same expected sample size ($\bar{N}_o$) 335 with futility stopping probability of 47%. This is because they use the same futility boundary and same sample size at the interim analysis for all three designs, while the efficacy stopping boundary has virtually no effect on sample size.

The R code for the simulation of the trial is presented below:

```
## Classical 1-Stage Design : Type-I error rate p10-p01-delNI=0
McNemarADwithSSR(alpha1=0.025, alpha2=0, beta1=0, p10=0.1, p01=0.175,
delNI=-0.075, nPairs1=322, nPairs2=0);
## Power for design with PF (rho=2), beta1=0.5 and SSR (Nmax>N0)
McNemarADwithSSR(alpha1=0.00625, alpha2=0.02173, beta1=0.5, p10=0.1,
p01=0.1, delNI=-0.075, nPairs1=161, nPairs2=161, nPairsMax=500);
```

Summary of Design

For sensitivity, totally 86 positive patients with one interim analysis will provide 95% power for the superiority test. The error-spending function for the stopping boundary is $\alpha\tau^2$, where τ is information time or sample-size fraction, and the futility stopping rule is $p_1 > \beta_1 = 0.5$. The design features a 43% early efficacy stopping probability if the alternative hypothesis is true and a 45% early futility stopping probability if the null hypothesis is true. The expected sample size is 68 and 67 under H_a and H_0, respectively, an 18% savings in comparison to 82 pairs for the classical design.

Given a 95% power for the sensitivity test and a 94% power for the specificity test, the two test statistics are assumed to be independent. The overall probability of getting an effectiveness claim for the diagnosis test (Method 2) is about 90%.

The stopping rules for sensitivity and specificity are the same. But sample-size reestimation is allowed for the design for specificity and the rules are specified as follows:

If the interim p-value for the sensitivity (specificity) test is $p_1 \leq 0.00625$, the null hypothesis for sensitivity (specificity) will be rejected. If the p-value for sensitivity (specificity) test is $p_1 > 0.5$, stop recruiting positive (negative) patients. If $0.5 \geq p_1 > 0.00625$, we continue to recruit positive (negative) patients and the sample size will be reestimated for negative patients based on a 90% conditional power. At the final analysis, if the p-value for the sensitivity (specificity) is $p_1 \leq 0.02173$, then the null hypothesis for sensitivity (specificity) will be rejected. In the end, if both null hypothesis tests for sensitivity and specificity are rejected, then the new diagnosis test (Method 2) will be claimed effective.

6.5 Trial with Incomplete Paired Data

6.5.1 *Mixture of Paired and Unpaired Data*

Missing data are a common occurrence in scientific research. In a survey, a lack of response constitutes missing data. In clinical trials, missing data can be caused by a patient's refusal to continue in a study, treatment failures, adverse events, or patient relocations. Missing data will complicate the data analysis. In many medical settings, missing data can cause difficulties in estimation and inference. In clinical trials, missing data can undermine randomization. The CHMP (Committee for Medicinal Product for Human use) CHMP guideline (2009) provide advices on how the presence of missing data in a confirmatory clinical trial should be addressed in a regulatory submission.

An example for missing in paired data would be either baseline or post-baseline measures missing for some patients. When multiple measures are taken from multiple locations in a body (e.g., left and right eyes), missing data often occur. In a 2×2 crossover trial, the outcomes are only present in one of the treatment periods for some patients. Case-control studies may also involve missing data. In such cases, the data from the trial become a mixture of paired and unpaired data. It is not uncommon that a meta-analysis involves a mixture of clustered and unclustered measures. Dealing with such a mixture of different data, a commonly used approach in clinical trial design and data analyses is to ignore the missing data or unpaired data. Such a treatment of data is obviously information wasting and not efficient at all.

According to Little and Rubin (2002), the mechanism of missingness can be classified into three different categories in terms of marginal probability distributions.

(1) If the probability of an observation being missing does not depend on observed or unobserved measurements, then the observation is classified as missing completely at random (MCAR).

(2) If the probability of an observation being missing depends only on observed measurements, then the observation is classified as missing at random (MAR). This assumption implies that the behavior (i.e., distribution) of the postdropout observations can be predicted from the observed values, and therefore that response can be estimated without bias using the observed data exclusively.

(3) When observations are neither MCAR nor MAR, they are classified as missing not at random (MNAR), i.e., the probability of an observation being missing depends on both observed and unobserved measurements.

Statistically, there is no way to know exactly whether missing is MCAR, MAR, or MNAR. However, we often believe MCAR/MAR can be a good approximation in certain situations.

6.5.2   *Minimum Variance Estimator*

Suppose in a clinical trial, each subject is intended to have two measures. However, in reality some subjects have only one measure and are missing the other. Therefore, the set of data becomes a mixture of paired and unpaired data.

Let $\hat{\delta}_p$ and $\hat{\delta}_u$ be the MLEs of the treatment differences between the two treatment groups for the paired and unpaired data, respectively. For the overall treatment difference we use the linear combination of the two:

$$\hat{\delta} = w_p \hat{\delta}_p + (1 - w_p)\hat{\delta}_u, \tag{6.11}$$

where the prefixed weight $w_p + w_u = 1$. Assuming MCAR or at least missing is not related to the treatment effect, then both estimators $\hat{\delta}_p$ and $\hat{\delta}_u$ are unbiased estimators of the treatment difference δ and $\hat{\delta}$, respectively.

We can choose the weights w_p and w_u so that variance $\sigma_{\hat{\delta}}^2$ is minimized, that is (Chang, 2015),

$$w_p = \frac{1}{1 + 2(1 - \rho)\frac{f_{1u}f_{2u}}{f_p(f_{1u}+f_{2u})}}, \tag{6.12}$$

where the total sample size $n = n_p + n_{1u} + n_{2u}$, $f_p = n_p/n$, $f_{iu} = n_{iu}/n$, (treatment $i = 1, 2$), and $\rho = $ the correlation coefficient between the matched pairs.

The minimum variance can be expressed as (Chang, 2015)

$$\sigma_\delta^2 = \frac{\sigma_*^2}{n}, \tag{6.13}$$

where the *equivalent variance* for the normal endpoint

$$\sigma_*^2 = \frac{2(1-\rho)\frac{1}{f_p}\left(\frac{1}{f_{1u}} + \frac{1}{f_{2u}}\right)}{2(1-\rho)\frac{1}{f_p} + \left(\frac{1}{f_{1u}} + \frac{1}{f_{2u}}\right)}\sigma_x^2. \tag{6.14}$$

The minimum-variance weight w_p has the following properties: (1) for paired data only, $n_u = 0$, and thus $w_p = 1$ and $w_u = 0$; (2) for independent data, $n_p = 0$, and thus $w_p = 0$ and $w_u = 1$; (3) when $\rho > 0$, $w_p > n_p/(n_p + n_u)$, i.e., a paired observation is weighted more than an unpaired observation; when $\rho < 0$, $w_p < n_p/(n_p + n_u)$, i.e., an unpaired observation is weighted more than a paired observation; as $\rho \to 0$, $w_p \to n_p/(n_p + n_u)$.

In (6.12), the correlation coefficient ρ should be determined independent of the current data. However, if ρ is (approximately) independent of $\hat{\delta}_u$ and $\hat{\delta}_p$ such as when n is large, the Pearson correlation coefficient, ρ, can be estimated from the data.

The two-sided $(1 - \alpha)100\%$ confidence interval for treatment difference δ is given by

$$w_p \delta_p + (1 - w_p)\delta_u \pm z_{1-\alpha/2}\frac{\sigma_*}{\sqrt{n}}. \tag{6.15}$$

For binary endpoint, a similar method is available (Chang, 2015).

6.5.3   *Retinal Disease Trial*

Visual acuity (VA) is often considered an outcome measure in clinical trials of retinal diseases. Sometimes the continuous VA letter score is dichotomized based on whether or not there has been a worsening (or gain) of ≥ 15 letters (equivalent to ≥ 3 lines). A study that contrasts these two approaches was carried out by Beck et. al (2007). Here we use continuous VA for the purpose of illustration of our method.

Suppose in a single group trial, we study the effect of a clinical intervention on the vision in patients with retinal disease. The Snellen eye chart is used with 20/20 being the normal visual acuity. A score of 20/100 means that, one can read at 20 feet a letter that people with "normal" vision can read at 100 feet. So at 20/100, one's vision acuity is very poor. Suppose the endpoint is the change from baseline in visual acuity. In the initial group sequential design without considering missing, we use the equivalent variance, $\sigma_*^2 = 2\sigma_x^2 (1 - \rho)$. However, there could be some missing observations for the clinical endpoint, i.e., some patients may have only a visual acuity score for one eye. If such missings are observed at interim analysis, the sample size will be adjusted using the common SSR approaches as described in Chapter 5, in which the effective size (normalized treatment difference) is calculated based on the observed treatment difference and equivalent variance σ_*^2.

Assume the treatment difference in visual acuity is $\delta = 0.1$ with a standard deviation $\sigma_x = 0.5$ and the correlation coefficient between baseline and post-baseline measures of same eyes, $\rho = 0.625$. For a 90% power and one-sided $\alpha = 0.025$, as a benchmark, the fixed sample size design requires about 200 subjects.

We now compare the classical design and the two different two-stage adaptive designs with blind SSR at the interim analysis. We initially estimated $\sigma_* = \sqrt{2}\sigma_x\sqrt{1 - \rho} = \sqrt{2}0.5\sqrt{1 - 0.625} = 0.433$ and treatment difference $\delta = 0.1$. The interim analysis is to be conducted at 50% information (100 subjects). For the blinded SSR, the interim analysis is used for SSR only without efficacy or futility stopping.

For unblinded SSR, we use a two-stage adaptive design with O'Brien-Fleming stopping boundary. The efficacy stopping boundary at p-value scale is 0.0026 and 0.024 for the interim and final analyses, respectively. The maximum sample size is 250, and interim analysis is performed on 100 patients' data.

Suppose that at the interim analysis, some patients have missing observations in one eye (for those who have missing endpoint measures in both eyes, we just need to replace those patients). Presumably, the interim data show $f_{1u} = 0.10$, $f_{2u} = 0.15$, $f_p = 0.75$, $\hat{\sigma}_x = 0.52$, $\hat{\rho} = 0.65$, from (6.14),

$$\hat{\sigma}_* = \sigma_x\sqrt{\frac{2(1-\rho)}{2(1-\rho)\frac{f_{1u}f_{2u}}{f_{1u}+f_{2u}}+f_p}} = 0.52\sqrt{\frac{2(1-0.65)}{2(1-0.65)\frac{0.10(0.15)}{0.10+0.15}+0.75}} = 0.489.$$

The simulations show that for the blinded SSR, the power for rejecting the null hypothesis is 92% with the average sample size 200. The early efficacy stopping probability is 32%. If the classical design is used with 200 subjects, the power will be 82% with $\delta = 0.1$ and $\hat{\sigma}_x = 0.489$. The simulation R code is presented below:

```
## Classical under Ha Power
ADwithIncompletePairs(alpha=0.025,                              alpha1=.025,
alpha2=0, beta1=0.5, sigma=0.433, NewSigma=0.433, N1=200, N2=0, Nmax =
200, u=0.1, cPower=0.9,)
ADwithIncompletePairs(alpha=0.025,                              alpha1=.025,
alpha2=0, beta1=0.5, sigma=0.489, NewSigma=0.489, N1=200, N2=0, Nmax =
200, u=0.1, cPower=0.9,)
```

Two-stage Adaptive Design with Blind SSR
ADwithIncompletePairs(alpha=0.025, alpha1=0.0026, alpha2=0.024, beta1=0.5, sigma=0.433, NewSigma=0.489, N1=100, N2=100, Nmin=200, Nmax = 250, u=0.1, cPower=0.9)

6.6 Trial with Coprimary Endpoints

6.6.1 *Introduction*

In the case of diseases of unknown etiology, where no clinical consensus has been reached on the single most important clinical efficacy endpoint, coprimary endpoints may be used. That is, when diseases manifest themselves in multidimensional ways, the efficacy requirement in a clinical trial is defined as meeting two or more endpoints simultaneously. Therefore, in an adaptive design of multiple endpoint trials, we have to deal with the multiplicity due to multiple endpoints and multiple analyses at different times. Cheng, et al. (2014) proved that the stopping boundaries from group sequential stopping boundaries with a single endpoint can be used directly without inflation or deflation of the type-I error and derived from the formulations for conditional power and power for group sequential design with multiple endpoints. The extension of the method to sample size reestimation design is also provided with illustrative examples (Cheng, 2014; Chang, 2014).

Hypotheses related to multiple coprimary endpoints have received a lot of attention in recent years (Meyerson et al., 2007). These problems are also called the reverse multiplicity problems. Examples of diseases where at least two primary endpoints may be of interest are (1) migraine accompanied by nausea and photophobia; (2) Alzheimer's disease assessed by Alzheimer's disease assessment scale–cognitive and clinician interview-based impression of change; (3) multiple sclerosis measured by relapse rate at 1 year and disability at 2 years; and (4) osteoarthritis evaluated by pain, patient global assessment, and quality of life. Hence, an efficacy in these diseases is evaluated with multiple endpoints. The study power may be considerably reduced in comparison with a single-endpoint problem, depending on the number of coprimary endpoints and the correlation(s) among the endpoints.

Consider that $X_1, X_2, ...X_N$ are independent random vectors drawn from the multivariate normal distribution with d dimensions $N_d(\boldsymbol{\mu}_d, \boldsymbol{\Sigma})$, where $\boldsymbol{\mu}_d = (\mu_1, \mu_2, ...\mu_d)'$. Without loss of generality, let $\boldsymbol{\Sigma} = (1-\rho)\boldsymbol{I}_d + \rho\boldsymbol{J}_d$. In this case, the covariance matrix of $\boldsymbol{X}$ and the correlation matrix are identical. We are interested in the following hypothesis:

$$H_0 : \mu_j \leq 0 \text{ for at least one } j \in (1, 2, \ldots, d) \tag{6.16}$$
$$H_a : \mu_j > 0 \text{ for all } j \in (1, 2, \ldots, d).$$

Table 6.7: Overall Power

Correlation	-0.8	-0.5	-0.2	0	0.2	0.5	0.8
Overall power	0.59	0.60	0.62	0.64	0.65	0.68	0.73

Note: Power for each individual endpoint = 80%.

Equivalently we can write the hypothesis test as

$$H_0 : \cup_{j=1}^d H_{0j} \text{ versus } H_a : \cap_{j=1}^d H_{aj}, \tag{6.17}$$

where $H_{0j} : \mu_j \leq 0$ and $H_{aj} : \mu_j > 0$. The test statistics for these individual endpoints are defined in a usual way: $Z_{Nj} = \sum_{i=1}^N X_{ij}/\sqrt{N}$. We reject H_{0j} if $Z_{Nj} \geq c$, the common critical value for all endpoints. Therefore we reject (6.16), and furthermore reject (6.17) if $Z_{Nj} \geq c$ for all j. It is straightforward to prove that for $\forall j$ and k, where $j, k = 1, 2, \ldots, d$, the covariance/correlation between the test statistics is the same as the covariance/correlation between the endpoints, i.e., $Corr(Z_{Nj}, Z_{Nk}) = \rho$ for $j \neq k$.

Consider a two-stage ($K = 2$) clinical trial with an interim analysis planned at information time $\tau = 0.5$ and the O'Brien-Fleming stopping boundaries are used; that is, the rejection boundaries are $z_{1-\alpha_1} = 2.80$ and $z_{1-\alpha_2} = 1.98$ at a one-sided level of significance $\alpha = 0.025$.

How the power varies as the ρ changes is shown in Table 6.7. For example, if we want to detect the effect size of 0.2 for each of the two normally distributed endpoints, 197 samples are needed for 80% power for each of the two endpoints. Using the group sequential design discussed above, the power with different correlations between endpoints is shown in Table 6.7. If the endpoints are more positively correlated, the overall power is higher.

6.6.2 *Group Sequential Trial*

For adaptive design, it is convenient to use simulation to determine the sample size or power.

Example 6.3: Power and Sample Size for Two-Arm Trial with Coprimary Endpoints

Suppose in a clinical trial, the standardized responses (mean divided by the standard deviation) for the two coprimary endpoints are estimated to be 0.2 and 0.25 for the test group and 0.005 and 0.015 for the control group. The correlation between the two endpoints is estimated to be $\rho = 0.25$. We use a two-stage group sequential design with O'Brien-Fleming boundary for efficacy stopping. The interim analysis will be performed at information time $\tau = 0.5$. To calculate the sample size for 85% overall power, we can invoke the R function with different sample size N until the power is close to 90%.

It turns out that N is 584 per group.

GSDwithCoprimaryEndpoints(mu11=0.2,mu12=0.25, mu21=0.005, mu22=0.015, rho=0.25, tau=0.5, c1=2.80, c2=1.98, N=584, nSims=10000)

6.7 Trial with Multiple Endpoints

Multiple-endpoint problems can arise in many different situations. For instance, when there is a single primary efficacy endpoint with one or more secondary endpoints, we try to claim the drug effect on primary and secondary endpoints; when there are two endpoints, at least one needs to be statistically significant to claim efficacy of the test drug; in a clinical trial we can use a surrogate endpoint for an accelerated approval and a clinically important endpoint for a full approval.

In this section, we will discuss adaptive designs for multiple-endpoint trials. Tang and Geller (1999) proposed the following test procedures to group sequential design with multiple endpoints.

Let $M = \{1, 2, \ldots, m\}$ be the set of indices for the m endpoints. Let F denote a nonempty subset of M and $H_{0,F}$ the null hypothesis $\mu_i = 0$ for $i \in F$. Let T_F be a test statistic for $H_{0,F}$. Consider a group sequential trial with K analyses. We use $T_{F,t}$ to indicate the dependence of T_F on the analysis time t. Let $\{\alpha_{F,t}, t = 1, 2, \ldots, K\}$ be a one-sided stopping boundary for testing $H_{0,F}$ such that $P_{H_{0,F}}\{T_{F,t} > \alpha_{F,t} \text{ for some } t\} \leq \alpha$. For a given vector u, let $I_u = \{i, \mu_i = 0\}$.

Tang and Geller proposed the following two procedures that preserve strong control of type-I errors.

Procedure 1

Step 1. Conduct interim analyses to test $H_{0,K}$, based on the stopping boundary $\{\alpha_{K,t}, t = 1, 2, \ldots, K\}$.

Step 2. When $H_{0,M}$ is rejected, say at time t^*, apply the closed testing procedure to test all the other hypotheses $H_{0,F}$ using T_{F,t^*} with α_{F,t^*} as the critical value.

Step 3. If any hypothesis is not rejected, continue the trial to the next stage, in which the closed testing procedure is repeated, with the previously rejected hypotheses automatically rejected without retesting.

Step 4. Repeat step 3 until all hypotheses are rejected or the last stage is reached.

We can modify procedure 2 slightly to obtain the following procedure.

Procedure 2

Step 1. Conduct interim analyses to test $H_{0,K}$, based on the group sequential boundary $\{\alpha_{K,t}, t = 1, 2, \ldots, K\}$.

Step 2. When $H_{0,M}$ is rejected, say at time t^*, apply the closed testing procedure to test all the other hypotheses $H_{0,F}$ using $T_{F,t^{**}}$ with $\alpha_{F,t^{**}}$ as the critical value for any predetermined IA time $t^{**} \leq t^*$.

Step 3. If any hypothesis is not rejected, continue the trial to the next stage, in which the closed testing procedure is repeated, with the previously rejected hypotheses automatically rejected without retesting.

Step 4. Repeat step 3 until all hypotheses are rejected or the last stage is reached.

Example 6.4 Three-Stage Adaptive Design for NHL Trial

A phase-III two-parallel group non-Hodgkin's lymphoma trial was designed with three analyses. The primary endpoint is progression-free survival (PFS); the secondary endpoints are (1) overall response rate (ORR) including complete and partial response and (2) complete response rate (CRR). The estimated median PFS is 7.8 months and 10 months for the control and test groups, respectively. Assume a uniform enrollment with an accrual period of 9 months and a total study duration of 23 months. The estimated ORR is 16% for the control group and 45% for the test group. The classical design with a fixed sample-size of 375 subjects per group will allow for detecting a 3-month difference in median PFS with 82% power at a one-sided significance level of $\alpha = 0.025$. The first interim analysis (IA) will be conducted on the first 125 patients/group (or total $N_1 = 250$) based on ORR. The objective of the first IA is to modify the randomization. Specifically, if the difference in ORR (test-control), $\Delta_{ORR} > 0$, the enrollment will continue. If $\Delta_{ORR} \leq 0$, then the enrollment will stop. If the enrollment is terminated prematurely, there will be one final analysis for efficacy based on PFS and possible efficacy claimed on the secondary endpoints. If the enrollment continues, there will be an interim analysis based on PFS and the final analysis of PFS. When the primary endpoint (PFS) is significant, the analyses for the secondary endpoints will be performed for the potential claim on the secondary endpoints. During the interim analyses, the patient enrollment will not stop. The number of patients at each stage is approximately as shown in Figure 6.1.

We use generalized Teng-Geller's procedure 2 with MINP for this trial as illustrated below.

The test statistic at the kth analysis is defined as:

$$z_{ik} = \sum_{j=1}^{k} w_{kj} \Phi^{-1}(1 - p_{ij}),$$

where the subscript i represents the ith endpoint, i.e., 1 for PFS, 2 for ORR, and 3 for CRR. p_{ij} is the stagewise p-value for the ith endpoint based on the

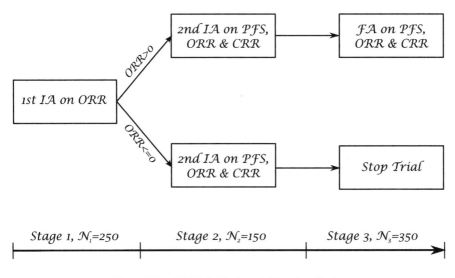

Figure 6.1: Multiple-Endpoint Adaptive Design

subsample from the jth stage.

$$w_{kj} = \sqrt{\frac{N_k}{\sum_{j=1}^{k} N_j}}.$$

The first IA does not intend to claim efficacy or futility, but modifies the enrollment (continues or not continues enrollment) based ORR. The stagewise test statistic is given by

$$z_{i1} = \Phi^{-1}(1 - p_{i1}).$$

At the 2nd IA, the test statistic is given by

$$Z_{i2} = 0.8\Phi^{-1}(1 - p_{i1}) + 0.6\Phi^{-1}(1 - p_{i2}). \tag{6.18}$$

If the trial continues after the 2nd IA, the test statistic at final analysis will be

$$Z_{i3} = 0.58\Phi^{-1}(1 - p_{i1}) + 0.45\Phi^{-1}(1 - p_{i2}) + 0.68\Phi^{-1}(1 - p_{i3}). \tag{6.19}$$

The OB-F stopping boundaries on the z-scale are $\alpha_1 = 3.490$, $\alpha_2 = 2.468$, $\alpha_3 = 2.015$ for stage 1, 2, and 3, respectively (Table 14.3). For simplicity, the same stopping boundaries are used for PFS, ORR, and CR.

Denote H_{0ij} the null hypothesis for the ith endpoint at j^{th} stage. The gatekeeper test procedure is described as follows: Construct the first hypothesis family as $F_1 = H_{011} \cap H_{012} \cap H_{013}$ for the PFS and similarly $F_2 = H_{021} \cap H_{022} \cap H_{023}$ for the ORR, and $F_3 = H_{031} \cap H_{032} \cap H_{033}$. F_1 is tested at level α; , if F_1 is not rejected, no further test will be tested. If

Table 6.8: MINP Based on Hypothetical p_{ik}

IA (k)	α_k	PFS		ORR		CRR	
		p_{1k}	z_{1k}	p_{2k}	z_{2k}	p_{3k}	z_{3k}
1	3.490	0.030	1.881	0.0002	3.60	0.10	1.281
2	2.468	0.034	2.600			0.12	1.730
3	2.015					0.065	2.300

F_1 is rejected, we further test F_2. If F_2 is not rejected, no further test will proceed. If F_2 is rejected, F_3 is tested. All tests will be conducted at the same level $\alpha = 0.025$. The (closed set) gatekeeper procedure ensures the strong control of FWE. Note that due to the correlation between PFS and ORR, we cannot just consider a two-stage weighting test statistic for PFS, even if the hypothesis test for PFS is not performed at the first IA.

Suppose at the first IA, the stagewise p-value for the primary endpoint (PFS) is $p_{11} = 0.030$ and the test statistic is $z_{11} = \Phi^{-1}(1 - p_{11}) = 1.881 < \alpha_1$, therefore the trial continues. At the second IA, the stagewise p-value $p_{12} = 0.034$, and the test statistic $z_{12} = 2.6$ is calculated from (6.18). Therefore the null hypothesis for PFS is rejected and the trial stops. Because the PFS is rejected, we can now test ORR. Suppose the stagewise p-value for ORR is $p_{21} = 0.002$ and $z_{21} = \Phi^{-1}(1 - p_{21}) = 3.60 > 3.490$; hence the null hypothesis for ORR is rejected. Because ORR is rejected, we can proceed with the test for CRR. Suppose that $p_{31} = 0.1$ and $z_{31} = 1.281 < \alpha_1$; $p_{32} = 0.12$ and $z_{32} = 1.73(< \alpha_2)$ from (6.18). Due to rejection of PFS at the second IA, the trial was stopped. However, the enrollment was not stopped during the interim analyses. At the time when the decision was made to stop the trial, 640 patients (approximately 320 per group) were enrolled. The gatekeeper procedure allows us to proceed to the third analysis of CRR. However, the rejection boundary needs to be recalculated through numerical integration or simulation based on the OB-F spending function. Based on the information time $\sqrt{640/750} = 0.923\,76$, the new rejection boundary is approximately $\alpha_{33}^* = 2.10$. Suppose that the observed $p_{33} = 0.065$ and the test statistic $z_{33} = 2.3$ is calculated from (6.19). Therefore CRR is also rejected. We can see that PFS, ORR, and CRR were all rejected, but at different times!!! The closed test project allows the rejections of different endpoints at different times (IAs) as illustrated in this example. The calculation is summarized in Table 6.8.

Chapter 7

Pick-the-Winners Design

7.1 Overview of Multiple-Arm Designs

An adaptive seamless phase-II/III design is one of the most attractive adaptive designs. A seamless adaptive design is a combination of traditional phase-II and phase-III trials. In seamless design, there is usually a so-called learning phase that serves the same purpose as a traditional phase-II trial, followed by a confirmatory phase that serves the same objectives as a traditional phase-III trial (Figure 7.1). Compared to traditional designs, a seamless design can reduce sample-size and time-to-market for a positive drug candidate.

A typical multiple-arm confirmatory adaptive design (often called drop-the-loser, drop-arm, or pick-the-winner design, adaptive dose-finding design, or phase-II/III seamless design) consists of two stages: a selection stage and a confirmation stage. For the selection stage, a randomized parallel design with several doses and a placebo group is employed for selection of doses. After the best dose is chosen (the winner), the patients of the selected dose group and placebo group continue to enter the confirmation stage. New patients will be recruited and randomized to receive the selected dose or placebo. The final analysis is performed with the cumulative data of patients from both stages (Chang, 2011; Maca et al., 2006).

As pointed out by Walton (2006), time between studies has multiple components: (1) analysis of observed data, (2) interpretation of analyzed results, (3) planning next study, (4) resource allocation, (5) selection of and agreements with investigators, (6) Institutional Review Board (IRB) submission and approval, and (7) other. In a seamless design, we move the majority of the "planning next study" to up-front; perform analysis at real time; and combine traditional two IRB submissions and approvals into one. Also, in seamless design there is one set of "selection of, agreements with, investigators" instead of two. Adaptive designs require adaptive or dynamic allocation of resources. At the end of traditional phase-IIb design, the analysis and interpretations of results are mainly performed by a sponsor and the "go and no-go"

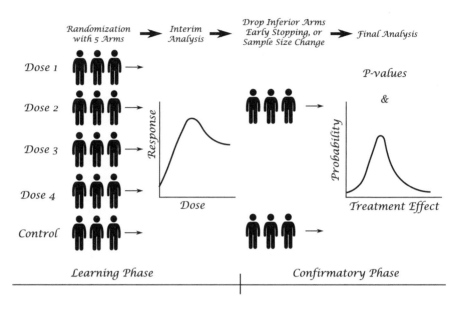

Figure 7.1:   Seamless Design

decision-making is fully made by a sponsor unless there are major safety concern. In seamless design, the traditional phase-IIb becomes the first phase of the seamless design and IDMC has a big inference on the decision. From that point of view, seamless design is less biased.

Huang, Liu, and Hsiao (2011) proposed a seamless design to allow prespecifying probabilities of rejecting the drug at each stage to improve the efficiency of the trial. Posch, Maurer, and Bretz (2011) described two approaches to control the type- error rate in adaptive designs with sample size reassessment and/or treatment selection. The first method adjusts the critical value using a simulation-based approach, which incorporates the number of patients at an interim analysis, the true response rates, the treatment selection rule, etc. The second method is an adaptive Bonferroni–Holm test procedure based on conditional error rates of the individual treatment–control comparisons. They showed that this procedure controls the type- error rate, even if a deviation from a preplanned adaptation rule or the time point of such a decision is necessary.

7.2   Pick-the-Winner Design

Suppose in a K-group trial, we define the global null hypothesis as $H_G : \mu_0 = \mu_1 = \mu_2 \cdots \mu_K$ and the hypothesis test between the selected arm (winner) and the control as

$$H_G : \mu_0 = \mu_s, \ s = \text{selected arm}. \tag{7.1}$$

Chang and Wang (2014) derive formulations for the two-stage pick-the-winner design with any number of arms. The design starts with all doses under consideration, at the interim analysis; the winner with the best response observed will continue to the second stage with the control group.

Suppose a trial starts with K dose groups (arms) and one control arm (arm 0). The maximum sample size for each group is N. The interim analysis will perform on N_1 independent observations per group, x_{ij} from $N\left(\mu_i, \sigma^2\right)$ $(i = 0, .., K; j = 1, \ldots, N_1)$. The active arm with maximum response at the interim analysis and the control arm will be selected and additional $N_2 = N - N_1$ subjects in each arm will be recruited. We denote by $\bar{x}_i$ the mean of the first N_1 observations in the ith arm $(i = 0, 1, ...K)$, and $\bar{y}_i$ the mean of the additional N_2 observations y_{ij} from $N\left(\mu_i, \sigma^2\right)$ $(i = 0, S; j = 1, \ldots, N_2)$. Here, arm S is the active arm selected for the second stage. Let $z_i = \frac{\bar{x}_i}{\sigma}\sqrt{N_1}$ and $\tau_i = \frac{\bar{y}_i}{\sigma}\sqrt{N_2}$, so that, under the H_G, t_i and τ_i are the standard normal distribution with pdf ϕ and cdf Φ, respectively.

Let's define the maximum statistic at the end of stage 1 as

$$Z_{(1)} = \max\left(t_1, t_2, \ldots, t_K\right). \tag{7.2}$$

At the final stage, using all data from the winner, we define the statistic

$$T^* = Z_{(1)}\sqrt{\tau} + \tau_s\sqrt{1-\tau}, \tag{7.3}$$

where $\tau = \frac{N_1}{N}$ is the information time at the interim analysis, and s is the selected arm.

The final test statistic is defined as

$$T = (T^* - t_0)/\sqrt{2}. \tag{7.4}$$

$$F_T(t) = \int_{-\infty}^{+\infty} \int_{-\infty}^{\infty} \left[\Phi\left(\frac{z - \tau_s\sqrt{1-\tau}}{\sqrt{\tau}}\right)\right]^K \phi(\tau_s)\phi\left(\sqrt{2}t - z\right) d\tau_s dz. \tag{7.5}$$

When the information time $\tau = 1$, (7.5) reduces to the c.d.f. for the Dunnett test:

$$F_T(t) = \int_{-\infty}^{\infty} [\Phi(z)]^K \phi\left(\sqrt{2}t - z\right) dz. \tag{7.6}$$

Table 7.1: Critical Value c_α for Classical Pick-the-Winner Design

Info Time τ	K						
	1	2	3	4	5	6	7
0.3	1.960	2.140	2.235	2.299	2.345	2.382	2.424
0.5	1.960	2.168	2.278	2.352	2.407	2.452	2.487
0.7	1.960	2.190	2.313	2.398	2.460	2.510	2.550

Note: 10,000,000 runs per scenario.

7.3   Stopping Boundary and Sample Size

Theoretically, the drop-arm design can reject H_0 at the interim (stage 1) analysis or reject H_0 at the final analysis. Here we will focus on the design that allows rejecting H_0 only at the final analysis. That is, if the observed test statistic $T_2 \geq c_\alpha$, the H_0 is rejected; otherwise, H_0 is not rejected. In such a case, the stopping boundary c_α can be determined using (7.6), that is, $F_{T_2}(c_\alpha) = 1 - \alpha$ for a one-sided significance level α. Numerical integration or simulation can be used to determine the stopping boundary and power. For $\tau = 0.5$, the numerical integrations (I use *Scientific Workplace*) give $c_\alpha = 2.352, 2.408, 2.451$, and 2.487 for $K = 4, 5, 6$, and 7, respectively, which are consistent with the results provided by the simulations in Table 7.1.

Example 7.1 Seamless Design of Asthma Trial

The objective of this trial in asthma patients is to confirm sustained treatment effect, measured as FEV1 change from baseline to the 1 year of treatment. Initially, patients are equally randomized to four doses of the new compound and a placebo. Based on early studies, the estimated FEV1 changes at week 4 are 6%, 12%, 13%, 14%, and 15% (with pooled standard deviation 18%) for the placebo (dose level 0) and dose levels 1, 2, 3, and 4, respectively. One interim analysis is planned when 60 per group or 50% of patients have the efficacy assessments. The interim analysis will lead to picking the winner (arm with best observed response). The winner and placebo will be used at stage 2. At stage 2, we will enroll additionally 60 patients per group in the winner and control groups.

The simulations show that the pick-the-winner design has 95% power with the total sample size of 420.

The typical simulation code is presented in the following:

```
## Determine Critical Value Z_alpha for 4+1 Arms Winner Design
mu=c(0,0,0,0)
WinnerDesign(nSims=1000000,NumOfArms=4, mu0=0, sigma=1, Z_alpha=2.352,
nStg1=60, nStg2=60)
## Determine Power for 4+1 Arms Winner Design
```

```
mu=c(0.12, 0.13, 0.14, 0.15)
WinnerDesign(nSims=100000,NumOfArms=4,        mu0=0.06,        sigma=0.18,
Z_alpha=2.352, nStg1=60, nStg2=60)
```

If we conduct the interim analysis earlier when 43 per group or 30% patients are enrolled (86 per group in the second stage), we only need 387 patients to achieve 95% power.

```
## Determine Critical Value Z_alpha for 4+1 Arms Winner Design
mu=c(0,0,0,0)
WinnerDesign(nSims=1000000,NumOfArms=4, mu0=0, sigma=1, Z_alpha=2.3,
nStg1=43, nStg2=86)
## Determine Power for 4+1 Arms Winner Design
mu=c(0.12, 0.13, 0.14, 0.15)
WinnerDesign(nSims=100000,NumOfArms=4,        mu0=0.06,        sigma=0.18,
Z_alpha=2.3, nStg1=43, nStg2=86)
```

For the same 5-arm trial, Dunnett design requires 510 subjects for 95% power. Here is the code to invoke the same R function with zero subjects for the second stage.

```
## Determine Critical Value Z_alpha for Dunnett Test
mu=c(0,0,0,0)
WinnerDesign(nSims=1000000,NumOfArms=4, mu0=0, sigma=1, Z_alpha=2.352,
nStg1=120, nStg2=0)
## Determine Power for Dunnett Test
mu=c(0.12, 0.13, 0.14, 0.15)
WinnerDesign(nSims=100000,NumOfArms=4,        mu0=0.06,        sigma=0.18,
Z_alpha=2.352, nStg1=120, nStg2=0)
```

7.4   Summary and Discussion

We have studied the seamless designs that allow for early dropping losers. Note that the efficiency of a seamless design is sensitive to the sample-size fraction or information time in the end of the learning phase. Therefore, simulations should be done to determine the best information time for the interim analysis.

Practically, the seamless trials require early efficacy readouts. This early efficacy assessment can be the primary endpoint for the trial or surrogate endpoint (biomarker). Because data analysis and interpretation allow exploration of richness of clinical data, the interim analysis should also include some variables other than the primary. Those analyses can be descriptive or hypothetical testing kinds. Seamless design can be also used for other situations such as a combination of phase-I and phase-II trials. Regarding the logistic issues in a seamless design, please see the papers by the PhRMA adaptive working group (Maca et al., 2006; Quinlan, Gallo, and Krams, 2006).

Chapter 8

The Add-Arms Design

8.1 Introduction

In the previous chapter we discussed the phases-II-III seamless designs, for which the type-I errors are strongly controlled. In contrast, there is another school of research on multiple-arm trials mainly for phase-II dose-finding studies, in which selecting target dose (dose schedule) such as minimum effective dose (MED) is the main purpose with a reasonable control of the type-I error. The MED can be defined as the dose where the mean efficacy outcome is equal to a certain target, with the placebo (or an active control) used as a reference. Mean efficacy is usually assumed to be nondecreasing with dose. Both efficacy and safety endpoints are often taken into consideration when selecting a dose for further studies in phase-III trials, because increasing the dose can result in both higher efficacy and increased adverse event rates. A common approach is to quantify efficacy and adverse event rate trade-off through a utility function that incorporates both efficacy and safety into a measure of overall clinical utility (Berry et al., 2001; Dragalin and Fedorov, 2006; Ivanova et al. 2009, 2012). Such a utility function is typically umbrella-shaped and the goal is to find a dose that maximizes the utility of the drug candidate. The objective in phase II can also be to test efficacy and adverse event rates at the estimated MED or the optimal dose against a control and recommend for further study in phase-III trials (Ivanova et al. 2012). Miller et al. (2007) investigated a two-stage strategy for a dose-ranging study that is optimal across several parametric models. Dragalin et al. (2008) investigated optimal two-stage designs for two correlated binary endpoints that follow a bivariate probit model. Bretz et al. (2005) studied the dose-finding methods under various dose-response scenarios including umbrella-shaped response curves. Ivanova et al. (2012) studied a Bayesian two-stage adaptive design for finding MED under the same set of dose-response curves and compared the section probability and power against uniform allocation method.

The seamless designs have some similarities to the phase-II dose-finding studies, but there are also differences. For example, the primary objective in a phase-II dose-finding might be to determine MED or ED90; therefore, the probability of selecting the target dose is the most important measure for evaluating a design, while type-I error control is secondary. In contrast, a seamless design focuses on the power of hypothesis testing with the strict control of the type-I error, but the probability of selecting best arm is secondary. Although the probability of selecting best arm and power are often closely related, they are not one-one mapping. The second difference might be in the endpoint: in a phase-II dose-finding study, the endpoint is usually a PD marker, but for the seamless design the endpoint is usually the primary efficacy endpoint for drug approval or its surrogate endpoint.

In this chapter, we will study the 3-stage add-arm adaptive designs proposed by Chang and Wang (2014). This method can be used for MED finding and phase-II-III seamless studies. In the pick-the-winner design, patients are randomized into all arms (doses) and at the interim analysis, inferior arms are dropped. Therefore, compared to the traditional dose-finding design, this adaptive design can reduce the sample size by not carrying over all doses to the end of the trial or dropping the losers earlier. However, all the doses have to be explored. For unimodal (including linear or umbrella) response curves, we proposed an effective dose-finding design that allows adding arms at the interim analysis. The trial design starts with two arms; depending on the response of the two arms and the unimodality assumption, we can decide which new arms to be added. This design does not require exploring all arms (doses) to find the best responsive dose; therefore it can further reduce the sample size from the drop-loser design.

The 3-stage add-arm design begins with only two active arms and the placebo (control) group. At the first interim analysis, more arms will be added depending on the observed responses of the two arms and assumption of unimodal (including monotonic and umbrella) response curve. The key idea of a drop-arm design is that "some inferior arms don't need to have a large exposure," whereas the central notion of the proposed 3-stage add-arm design is that "some inferior arms don't have to be exposed at all" when the response is unimodal (umbrella-shaped).

For convenience, we define the global null hypothesis as $H_G : \mu_0 = \mu_1 = \mu_2 = \cdots = \mu_K$ and the hypothesis test between the selected arm (winner) and the control as

$$H_0 : \mu_0 = \mu_s, \ s = \text{selected arm}. \tag{8.1}$$

8.2   The Add-Arm Design

8.2.1   *Design Description*

The add-arm design is a three-stage adaptive design, in which we can use interim analyses and the unimode-response property to determine which doses cannot (unlikely) be the arm with best response–thus no exposure to those doses is necessary. Let's take a 4+1 arm design as an example to illustrate the key idea behind the add-arm design.

In the 4+1 arm design, there are $K = 4$ dose levels (active arms) and a placebo arm (dose level 0). Theoretically, if we know dose 2 has a larger response than dose 3, then we know, by the unimode-response assumption, that the best response arm can be either dose 1 or 2, but not dose 4. Therefore, we don't need to test dose 4 at all. Similarly, if we know dose 3 has a larger response than dose 2, then we know, by the unimode-response assumption, that the best response arm can be either dose 4 or 3, but not dose 1. Therefore, we don't need to test dose 1 at all. The problem is that we don't know the true responses for doses 2 and 3. We have to find them out based on the observed responses. Of course, we want the observed rates to reflect the true responses with high probability, which mean the sample size cannot be very small.

We are now ready to fully describe the three-stage 4+1 add-arm design (Figure 8.1). At the first stage, randomize subjects in two active and the placebo groups. The second stage is the add-arm stage, at which we determine which arm to be added based on the observed data from the first stage and the unimodal property of the response curve. At the third or final stage, more subjects will be added to the winner arm and the placebo. The randomization is specified as follows:

- Stage 1: Assign $2.5N_1$ subjects in arms 2, 0, and 3 using randomization ratio $N_1 : N_1/2 : N_1$.
- Stage 2: If $t_2 > t_3$, assign $1.5N_1$ subjects in arms 0 and 1 using a $N_1/2 : N_1$ randomization. If $t_2 \leq t_3$, assign $1.5N_1$ subjects in arm 0 and 4 using a $N_1/2 : N_1$ randomization.
- Stage 3: (a) If $t_2 > t_3$ and $t_2 - t_1 > c_R$, select arm 2 as the winner; otherwise, select arm 1 as the winner. If $t_2 \leq t_3$ and $t_3 - t_4 > c_R$, select arm 3 as the winner; otherwise, select arm 4 as the winner. (b) Assign $2N_2$ subjects in arms 0 and the winner arm using $N_2 : N_2$ randomization.

Therefore, there will be $4N_1 + 2N_2$ total subjects. In the final analysis for the hypothesis test, we will use the data from $N_1 + N_2$ subjects in the winner and $N_1 + N_2$ subjects in arm 0.

One may have noticed that we use a $N_1/2 : N_1 : N_1$ randomization instead of a $N_1 : N_1 : N_1$ randomization. This is because the imbalanced

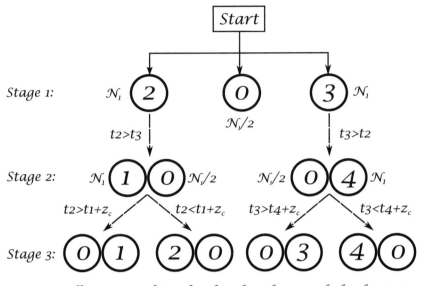

Enroll N_2 more subjects for the selected arm and placebo at stage 3
N_1+N_2 subjects in the selected arm and placebo for the final analysis

Figure 8.1: The 4+1 Add-Arm Design

randomization can keep the treatment blinding and balance the confounding factors at both stages. If N_1 placebo subjects all randomized in the first stage, then at the second stage all N_1 subjects will be assigned to the active group without randomization, thus unblinding the treatment and potentially imbalancing some (baseline) confounding factors.

A key question is how to determine the constant c_R. Before we discuss it, it is convenient to define the term "selection probability," that is, the probability of selecting a dose as the preferred dose for the next stage of the adaptive trial. We noticed that if $c_R = 0$, the design becomes a three-stage pick-the-winner (or drop–the-loser) design, in which the active arm with the maximum observed response at the current stage is picked as the winner. The problem with this is that the selection probability will be skewed when the response curve is flat. Particularly, the selection probabilities of doses 1, 2, 3, and 4 are 1/6, 2/6, 2/6, and 1/6, respectively, when in fact all doses have the same response. The real issue with this uneven selection probability is that when, for example, dose 1 has a better response than dose 2, there could still be a large probability of selecting dose 2 or 3 than dose 1 as the winner.

Therefore, we have to force the selection probability equal (or at least approximately equal) for all doses when H_G is true. To this end, we want the selection probability at the second stage to be $1/4$ under H_G, i.e.,

$$P(t_2 - t_1 > c_R \cap t_2 > t_3; H_G) = 1/4. \tag{8.2}$$

For the normal distribution, the selection probability is given by (see Appendix A)

$$P(t_2 - t_1 > c_R \cap t_2 > t_3; H_G) = \int_{-\infty}^{\infty} \Phi(x - c_R)\phi(x)\Phi(x)\,dx. \tag{8.3}$$

To summarize, the two key ideas in this design are: (1) using the unimode-response property to determine which arms not to explore, and (2) determining the rule (c_R) for picking the winner so that the selection probabilities for all active arms are (at least approximately) equal under a flat response curve.

8.2.2 *Controlling Selection Probability and Type-I Error*

The first step is to determine the threshold c_R and critical value for rejection of H_G, which can be determined using simulations. The results are presented in Table 8.1 for the 4+1 add-arm designs with one-sided $\alpha = 0.025$. Each set of results is based on 10,000,000 simulation runs. In Table 8.1, we have also presented the proportion of the α spent on each arm. For instance, for the 4+1 design, under H_G, among all rejections, 20% rejections with the winner being arm 1; and 30% with the winner being arm 2; 30% with the winner being arm 3; and 20% with the winner being arm 4. We can see that c_R is so determined that it gives equal chance to select any dose when all doses have the same effect, but the α spent on each arm is different. This desirable feature allows one to use the prior knowledge to spend more alpha on the promising doses to achieve more efficient (powerful) design. We further noticed that it's sometimes desirable to have particular α-spending among doses by modifying the c_R slightly and the information time τ. When this occurs, the stopping boundaries should be modified accordingly so that the familywise error is controlled. The values c_R and c_α for the add-arm designs with $\alpha = 0.025$ and $\tau = 0.5$ are presented in Table 8.1.

Since these stopping boundaries are determined based on normality or large sample size assumption, we want to know how well they can be applied to the case of small sample size. For sample size $N_1 = N_2 = 30$, the error rate is 0.0278, a small inflation from 0.025. Based on simulations (1,000,000 runs), for sample size $N_1 = N_2 = 100$, the inflation is negligible or within the random fluctuation by the simulation. When the sample size is smaller than 30, the critical value can be determined by simulations. It is a good practice to check type-I error rate using simulation before running the power simulations. Note that for sample size 30 per group in a classical two-arm

Table 8.1: c_R, c_α ($\alpha = 0.025$)

Selection Method	τ	c_R	c_α
Fair	0.3	0.5565	2.208
Skew	0.3	0	2.225
Fair	0.5	0.5565	2.267
Skew	0.5	0	2.275
Fair	0.7	0.5565	2.300
Skew	0.7	0	2.312

design, the type-I error will be inflated from 0.025 to 0.0274 if using normal distribution approximation for the univariate t-test.

Invoke the 4+1 add-arm design function:

```
mu=c(0,0,0,0)
FourPlus1AddArmDesign(nSims=100000, N1=100, N2=100, c_alpha = 2.267,cR = 0.55652, mu0=0, sigma=1)
mu=c(0.4,0.58,0.7,0.45)
FourPlus1AddArmDesign(nSims=10000, N1=116, N2=116, c_alpha = 2.267,cR = 0.55652, mu0=0.35, sigma=0.9)
```

8.3   Clinical Trial Examples

8.3.1   *Phase-II Dose-Finding Designs*

For phase-II dose-finding trials, we need to define response value at the minimum effective dose (MED), μ_{MED}, which will be used to define the utility function:

$$U = \frac{1}{(\mu_i - \mu_{MED})^2},\tag{8.4}$$

where μ_i is the response in arm i. Using this utility, we can convert the problem of finding the MED to the problem of finding the dose with the maximum utility U because at or near the MED, the maximum of U is achieved. However, to prevent a numerical overflow in the simulation, we have implemented the utility using

$$U = \frac{1}{(\hat{\mu}_i - \mu_{MED})^2 + \varepsilon},\tag{8.5}$$

where $\varepsilon > 0$ is a very small value (e.g., 0.00000001) introduced to avoid a numerical overflow when the observed $\hat{\mu}_i = \mu_{MED}$.

Example 8.1: Phase-II Dose-Finding Trial

Anemia is a condition in which the body does not have enough healthy red blood cells. Iron helps make red blood cells. When the body does not have enough iron, it will make fewer red blood cells. This is called iron deficiency anemia (IDA). IDA is the most common form of anemia (Locker, et al., 1997). The majority of IDA is linked to menstrual blood loss, pregnancy, postpartum blood loss, GI bleeding, cancer, or chronic kidney disease (CKD) (Baker, 2000).

The hypothetical drug candidate, FXT, is an IV drug candidate for treating patients with IDA. Serious hypersensitivity reactions and cardiovascular events among others are the potential main safety concerns regarding the use of IV iron products. Therefore, the goal is to find the minimum effective dose (MED). It was hypothetically determined that 0.5g/dL is the minimal clinical meaningfully in Hg change from baseline.

Suppose 4 active doses (200 mg, 300 mg, 400 mg, 500 mg) are to be investigated. The primary endpoint is hemoglobin (Hg) change from baseline to week 5, which is an objective measure in the lab. Assume an E_{max} model with responses (Hg change from baseline to week 5) of 0, 0.34, 0.68, 0.76, and 0.78 g/dL for the placebo and 4 active doses with a common standard deviation of 1.6. Because Hg is objectively measured in the lab, the placebo effect, if any, will be minimal.

The target response of MED is determined to be 0.7 g/dL, which is somewhat higher than the minimal clinically meaningful difference 0.5 g/dL. This is because if we define MED with response 0.5, then there is a 50% probability that the observed response of the MED will be less than 0.5 g/dL, regardless of sample size or power. We want the probability of observing response at the target MED > 0.5 much higher than 50%.

To use the add-arm and drop-arm designs, we first need to define the unimodal utility function using (8.5) so that the MED-finding problem becomes the problem of finding the dose with the maximum utility. The performances of the add-arm and drop-arm designs are evaluated using simulations. The results are presented in Table 8.2.

For the $4 + 1$ add-arm design with one-sided $\alpha = 0.025$, the critical value $c_\alpha = 2.267$, $c_R = 0.55652$, $N_1 = 45$, $N_2 = 90$, and power $= 90\%$, the total sample size required is 360. For the $4 + 1$ drop-arm design with $c_\alpha = 2.35$,

Table 8.2: Selection Probability and Sample Size: AA and DA Designs

Design method	d_1	d_2	d_3	d_4	Sample size
	200 mg	400 mg	500 mg	300 mg	
Add-arm design	0.074	0.436	0.326	0.164	360
Drop-arm design	0.102	0.319	0.296	0.283	432

$N_1 = 48$, $N_2 = 96$, and power = 90%, the total required sample size is 432. The add-arm design can save 72 subjects or 17% sample size from the drop-arm design. In both methods, the type-I error rates are below 2.5% according to 1,000,000 simulation runs.

8.3.2　*Phase-II-III Seamless Designs*

Example 8.2: Phase-II-III Asthma Trial

This hypothetical phase-II-III seamless design is motivated by an actual asthma clinical development program. AXP is a second generation compound in the class of asthma therapies known as 5-LO inhibitors, which block the production of leukotrienes. Leukotrienes are major mediators of the inflammatory response. The company's preclinical and early clinical data suggested that the drug candidate has potential for an improved efficacy and is well tolerated under the total dose of 1600 mg.

The objective of the multicenter seamless trial is to evaluate the effectiveness (as measured by FEV1) of oral AXP in adult patients with chronic asthma. Patients were randomized to one of five treatment arms, arm 0 (placebo), arm 1 (daily dose of 200 mg for 6 weeks), arm 2 (daily dose of 400 mg for 4 weeks), arm 3 (daily dose of 500 mg 3 weeks), and arm 4 (daily dose of 300 mg for 5 weeks). Since the efficacy is usually dependent on both AUC and C_{max} of the active agent it is difficult to judge at the design stage exactly which dose-schedule combination will be the best. However, based on limited data and clinical judgment it might be reasonable to assume that the following dose sequence might show a unimodal (umbrella) response curve: arm 1, arm 2, arm 3, and arm 4. The dose responses are estimated to be 8%, 13%, 17%, 16%, and 15% for the placebo and the four active arms with a standard deviation of 26%.

We compare the 4+1 add-arm design against the drop-arm design. A total sample size of 600 subjects ($N_1 = N_2 = 100$) for the add-arm design will provide 89% power. We have also tried other different dose sequences, including wavelike sequence; the simulation results show that the power ranges from 88% to 89%, except for the linear response, which provides 86% power. Comparing the drop-arm design, 602 subjects ($N_1 = N_2 = 86$) will provide only 84% power, regardless of dose sequence. Given the good safety profile, the selection probability is much less important than the power. Thus, the slight difference in selection probability is not discussed here.

8.3.3　*Phase-IV Postmarketing Study*

Example 8.3: Phase-IV Oncology Trial

Multiple myeloma is a cancer of plasma cells, a type of white blood cell present in bone marrow. Plasma cells normally make antibodies to fight infections. In multiple myeloma, a group of plasma cells (myeloma cells) becomes cancerous and multiplies, raising the number of plasma cells to a higher than normal level. Health problems caused by multiple myeloma can affect one's bones, immune system, kidneys, and red blood cell count. Myeloma develops in 1–4 per 100,000 people per year. There is no cure for multiple myeloma, but treatments are available that slow its progression.

The chemical compound V was a newly approved third line (hypothetical) drug for multiple myeloma in addition to several other drugs (labeled X, Y, Z, ...) available for the same disease indication. An investigator wants to know which of the following drug combinations will provide the most benefit to the patients: $V+X$, $V+Y$, $V+Z$, or $V+X+Y$. The reasons for such combinations are that the mechanism of action of V is different from X, Y, and Z, while X and Y are similar but with some difference in the mechanism. However, X and Y are very similar to Z in the mechanics of action; thus to combine them $(X + Z$ or $Y + Z)$ will not increase the response. To seek the company's sponsorship, the investigator has looked into different designs: the drop-arm design and the add-arm design. For this phase-IV trial, it is determined that the surrogate endpoint of tumor size reduction (partial response + complete response rate) is the primary endpoint. Complete response (CR) is defined as 100% M-protein reduction and partial response (PR) is more than 50% reduction in tumor size.

The standard treatment (S) has a response rate of 42%. The estimated rates for $V + X$, $V + Y$, $V + Z$, and $V + X + Y$ are 50%, 54%, 57%, and 60%, respectively. Given such estimates, the $4 + 1$ add-arm design is considered and the arms are arranged as follows: arm 1: $V + X$, arm 2: $V + Y$, arm 3: $V + X + Y$, and arm 4: $V + Z$ with response sequence: 50%, 54%, 60%, and 57%. With the large sample size assumption, the standard deviation is estimated (somewhat conservatively) to be $\sigma = \sqrt{p(1-p)} \approx 0.5$ for all the arms, where p is the tumor response rate.

We can see that in this setting, both the correct selection probability and power are important measures of a trial design. For a total sample size of 300 $(N_1 = N_2 = 100)$ and $\alpha = 0.025$, the 4+1 add-arm design will provide 88% power and correct selection probability for the best arm is 47%. For the same total sample size $(N_1 = 80$ and $N_2 = 140)$, the power of the add-arm design increases to 89% but correct selection probability reduces to 44%. Given the main objective of the trial is to recommend a best drug combination therapy, the first design with $N_1 = N_2 = 100$ seems a better design.

We know that the constant c_R can also dramatically affect the selection probability and power. For example, if we change c_R from 0.55652 to 0, the correct selection probability will change from 47% to 59% and power will change from 88% to 90%. If the c_R is changed further to -1, the correct selection probability will be 74% and power 90%. However, such a deviation (to a more extreme value) from the default value $c_R = 0.5565$ could negatively affect the selection probability and power if the response pattern is estimated very inaccurately.

Considering all these factors, the add-arm design with $N_1 = N_2 = 100$ and $c_R = 0$ is recommended. To compare, for the same 90% power, the drop-arm design requires 700 ($N_1 = N_2 = 100$) subjects with the correct selection probability of 58%. Thus the add-arm design requires 100 fewer subjects or 17% savings in sample size from the drop-arm design in this scenario.

8.4   Extension of Add-Arms Designs

8.4.1   *Design Description*

The 4+1 add-arm design can be extended to designs, for example, (1) with more arms, (2) allowing early rejections, and (3) with interim futility stopping (if the nonbinding futility rule is used, the stopping boundary remains unchanged).

The 5+1 Add-Arm Design

The 5+1 add-arm design consists of 5 active arms and placebo (control) arm (Figure 8.2). The randomization and dose selection rules are specified as

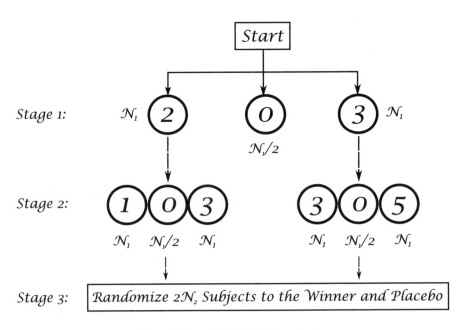

Figure 8.2:   The 5+1 Add-Arm Design

follows:

- Stage 1: Assign $2.5N_1$ subjects to arms 2, 0, and 4 using randomization ratio $N_1 : N_1/2 : N_1$.
- Stage 2: If $t_2 > t_4$, assign $2.5N_1$ subjects in arms 1, 0 and 3 using a $N_1 : N_1/2 : N_1$ randomization. If $t_2 \leq t_4$, assign $2.5N_1$ subjects in arms 3, 0, and 5 using a $N_1 : N_1/2 : N_1$ randomization.
- Stage 3: (a) If $t_2 > t_4$ and $\max(t_2, t_3) - t_1 < c_R$, select arm 1 as the winner; otherwise, select arm 2 or 3 as the winner depending on which has a larger observed response. If $t_2 \leq t_4$ and $\max(t_3, t_4) - t_5 < c_R$, select arm 5 as the winner; otherwise, select arm 4 or 3 as the winner depending on which has a larger response. (b) Assign $2N_2$ subjects in arm 0 and the winner arm using $N_2 : N_2$ randomization.

Therefore, there will be totally $5N_1 + 2N_2$ subjects. In the final analysis for the hypothesis test, we will use the data from $N_1 + N_2$ subjects in the winner and $N_1 + N_2$ subjects in arm 0.

The 6+1 Add-Arm Design

The 6+1 add-arm design consists of 6 active arms and placebo (control) arm (Figure 8.3). The randomization and dose selection rules are specified as follows:

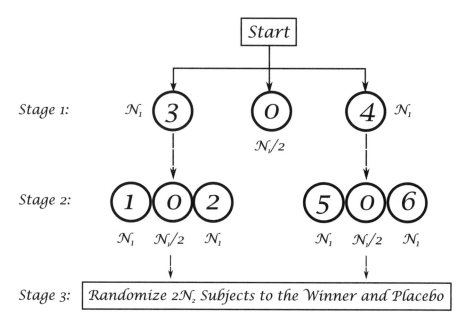

Figure 8.3: The 6+1 Add-Arm Design

- Stage 1: Assign $2.5N_1$ subjects in arms 3, 0, and 4 using randomization ratio $N_1 : N_1/2 : N_1$.
- Stage 2: If $t_3 > t_4$, assign $2.5N_1$ subjects in arms 1, 0, and 2 using a $N_1 : N_1/2 : N_1$ randomization. If $t_3 \leq t_4$, assign $2.5N_1$ subjects in arms 5, 0, and 6 using a $N_1 : N_1/2 : N_1$ randomization.
- Stage 3: (a) If $t_3 > t_4$ and $t_3 - \max(t_1, t_2) > c_R$, select arm 3 as the winner; otherwise, select arm 1 or 2 as the winner depending on which has a larger observed response. If $t_3 \leq t_4$ and $t_4 - \max(t_5, t_6) > c_R$, select arm 4 as the winner; otherwise, select arm 5 or 6 as the winner depending on which has a larger response. (b) Assign $2N_2$ subjects in arm 0 and the winner arm using $N_2 : N_2$ randomization.

Therefore, there will be total $5N_1 + 2N_2$ subjects. In the final analysis for the hypothesis test, we will use the data from $N_1 + N_2$ subjects in the winner and $N_1 + N_2$ subjects in arm 0.

The 7+1 Add-Arm Design

The 7+1 add-arm design consists of 7 active arms and placebo (control) arm (Figure 8.4). The randomization and dose selection rules are specified as follows:

- Stage 1: Assign $2.5N_1$ subjects in arms 3, 0, and 5 using randomization ratio $N_1 : N_1/2 : N_1$.

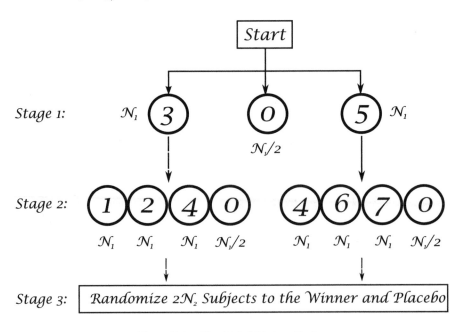

Figure 8.4:   The 7+1 Add-Arm Design

- Stage 2: If $t_3 > t_5$, assign $3.5N_1$ subjects in arms 1, 2, 4, and 0 using a $N_1 : N_1 : N_1 : N_1/2$ randomization. If $t_3 \leq t_5$, assign $3.5N_1$ subjects in arms 4, 6, 7, and 0 using a $N_1 : N_1 : N_1 : N_1/2$ randomization.
- Stage 3: (a) If $t_3 > t_5$ and $\max(t_1, t_2) > \max(t_3, t_4) - c_R$, select arm 1 or 2 as the winner depending on which has a larger response; otherwise, select arm 3 or 4 as the winner depending on which has a larger response. If $t_3 \leq t_5$ and $\max(t_7, t_6) > \max(t_5, t_4) - c_R$, select arm 7 or 6 as the winner; otherwise, select arm 5 or 4 as the winner depending on which has a larger response. (b) Assign $2N_2$ subjects in arm 0 and the winner arm using a $N_2 : N_2$ randomization.

Therefore, a sample size of $6N_1 + 2N_2$ subjects is required. In the final analysis for the hypothesis test, we will use the data from $N_1 + N_2$ subjects in the winner and $N_1 + N_2$ subjects in the arm 0.

8.4.2 *Stopping Boundary and Selection Probability*

The first step is to determine the threshold c_R and critical value for rejection of H_G, which can be determined using simulations. The results are presented in Table 8.3 for the 4+1 to 7+1 add-arm designs with one-sided $\alpha = 0.025$. Each set of results is based on 10,000,000 simulation runs. In Table 8.3, we have also presented the proportion of the α spent on each arm. For instance, for the 4+1 design, under H_G, among all rejections, 20% rejections with the winner being arm 1, 30% with the winner being arm 2, 30% with the winner being arm 3, and 20% with the winner being arm 4. We can see that c_R is so determined that it gives equal chance to select any dose when all doses have the same effect, but the α spent on each arm is different. This desirable feature allows one to use the prior knowledge to spend more alpha on the promising doses to achieve more efficient (powerful) design. We further noticed that it's sometimes desirable to have particular α-spending among doses by modifying the c_R slightly and the information time τ. When this occurs, the stopping boundaries should be modified accordingly so that the familywise error is controlled. The values c_R and c_α for the add-arm designs with $\alpha = 0.025$ and $\tau = 0.5$ are presented in Table 8.3.

Table 8.3: c_R, c_α and Percent of α Spent ($\alpha = 0.025$, $\tau = 0.5$)

Design	c_R	c_α	(Virtual) Dose Level						
			1	2	3	4	5	6	7
4+1	0.5565	2.267	20.0	30.0	30.0	20.0	—	—	—
5+1	0.5215	2.343	15.8	22.8	22.8	22.8	15.8	—	—
6+1	0.5009	2.341	14.4	14.4	21.2	21.2	14.4	14.4	—
7+1	0.4800	2.397	11.7	12.0	17.2	17.2	17.2	12.0	11.7

Table 8.4: Responses for Difference Response Curves

Design	Curve Name	0	1	2	3	4	5	6	7
4+1	Linear	0	0.1	0.2	0.3	0.4	—	—	—
	UM1	0	0.1	0.2	0.4	0.3	—	—	—
	UM2	0	0.1	0.4	0.3	0.2	—	—	—
5+1	Linear	0	0.08	0.16	0.24	0.32	0.40	—	—
	UM1	0	0.08	0.16	0.24	0.40	0.32	—	—
	UM2	0	0.08	0.16	0.40	0.32	0.24	—	—
	UM3	0	0.08	0.40	0.32	0.24	0.16	—	—
6+1	Linear	0	0.067	0.133	0.200	0.267	0.333	0.400	—
	UM1	0	0.067	0.133	0.200	0.267	0.400	0.333	—
	UM2	0	0.067	0.133	0.200	0.400	0.333	0.267	—
	UM3	0	0.067	0.133	0.400	0.333	0.267	0.200	—
	UM4	0	0.067	0.400	0.333	0.267	0.200	0.133	—
7+1	Linear	0	0.057	0.114	0.171	0.229	0.286	0.343	0.400
	UM1	0	0.057	0.114	0.171	0.229	0.286	0.400	0.343
	UM2	0	0.057	0.114	0.171	0.229	0.400	0.343	0.286
	UM3	0	0.057	0.114	0.171	0.400	0.343	0.286	0.229
	UM4	0	0.057	0.114	0.400	0.343	0.286	0.229	0.171
	UM5	0	0.057	0.400	0.343	0.286	0.229	0.171	0.114

8.4.3 Comparison of Power

To compare the power of the add-arm designs against the drop-arm designs, various dose-response curves are considered. The different response curves are obtained by switching the sequence of the doses (Table 8.4). For the drop-arm design, the dose sequence is irrelevant as far as the power is concerned. However, for the add-arm design, a different dose sequence implies a different test order.

For the drop-arm design, there are two stages and the sample size (per group) ratio at the first stage to the second stage is $N_1/N_2 = 1$ or information time $\tau_1 = \tau_2 = 0.5$. From the numerical integrations with $\tau_1 = \tau_2 = 0.5$, the rejection boundaries for the 4+1, 5+1, 6+1, and 7+1 drop-arm designs are 2.352, 2.408, 2.451, and 2.487, respectively.

Based on 1,000,000 simulation runs for each scenario, the sample size and power are presented in Table 8.5 for the add-arm and drop-arm (DA) designs for different response curves. For the each add-arm design ($\tau_1 = \tau_2 = 0.5$), we also presented the average power over different response curves. For the drop-arm design, the dose sequence is irrelevant; thus the power is identical for all the response curves.

Table 8.5: Power (%) Comparisons

Design	N_{max}	Response Curve						Average Power	DA Power
		Linear	UM1	UM2	UM3	UM4	UM5		
4+1	700	90.2	95.3	96.6	—	—	—	94.0	90.0
5+1	700	90.5	92.7	92.8	94.0	—	—	92.5	89.8
6+1	700	81.0	81.0	91.8	94.0	89.2	—	87.4	85.8
7+1	700	82.2	82.2	88.6	89.4	91.1	87.3	86.8	81.7

As mentioned previously, the total sample size N_{max} is $(K+1)N_1+2N_2$ for the $K+1$ drop-arm design, $4N_1+2N_2$ for the 4+1 add-arm design, $5N_1+2N_2$ for the 5+1 add-arm and the 6+1add-arm designs, and $6N_1+2N_2$ for the 7+1 add-arm design.

From the results, we can see that the add-arm designs generally provide a higher average power (2%–5% higher) than drop-arm designs. All add-arm designs (except the 6+1 design) provide higher power than the corresponding drop-arm designs under all different response curves. The reason that the 6+1 design is not always higher than the drop-arm design is because it is difficult to identify the better arm in the first stage when their responses are similar in the two arms at the first stage. We also want to point out that when there are larger response differences between arms the linear response arrangement is very unlikely to happen since if one is so unsure about response curve (i.e., thought response was umbrella-shaped but it is actually linear with a large slope), one should not assume the unimodality at all. On the other hand, if one knew the monotonic response (even with the slope quite flat), one would have rearranged the dose sequence to make it more likely to be umbrella-shaped.

In addition, we can compare the drop-arm and the add-arm designs under some scenarios that are suspected to be unfavorable to the proposed add-arm design: (1) when the dose responses of the two arms at the first stage are the same and (2) when the response curve is wavelike, but the fluctuation is small. The first dose response curve (named flat in Table 8.6) with an equal response for the two doses at the first stage is $(0.2, 0.2, 0.3, 0.45, 0.3, 0.25)$ for dose sequence $(d_0, d_1, d_2, d_3, d_4, d_5)$ and the second wavelike response curve is $(0.2, 0.2, 0.4, 0.38, 0.42, 0.45)$ for the same dose sequence. We compare the 5+1 add-arm design and 5+1 drop-arm design in terms of power and selection probability. The simulations are based on the standard deviation of 1.5, total sample size of 3,500, and one-sided α of 0.025. The simulation results are presented in Table 8.6. From the results we see that the add-arm is still superior to the drop-arm design in terms of power and correct selection probabilities. The reason is that when the response is wavelike but the waves are small, it is unnecessary to have many arms.

Table 8.6: Comparison of Power and Selection Probability

Response	Design Method	N_1/N_2	d_1	d_2	d_3	d_4	d_5	Power
Flat	Add-arm design	500/500	0.00	0.05	0.89	0.05	0.01	0.88
	Drop-arm design	438/438	0.00	0.06	0.87	0.06	0.02	0.82
Wave	Add-arm design	500/500	0.00	0.32	0.14	0.21	0.32	0.91
	Drop-arm design	438/438	0.00	0.18	0.12	0.26	0.45	0.89

This kinds of settings may reflect the following practical scenarios. For some disease indications, such as cardiovascular and oncology, the primary efficacy endpoint and the primary safety endpoint are consistent. For example, the composite endpoint of death and MI in 30 days is often the efficacy and safety endpoints for cardiovascular studies. Survival or death is often the efficacy and safety endpoint for cancer trials. In such cases, the dose-responses are usually monotonic but we can rearrange the dose sequence so that the responses become a unimodal or an umbrella-shaped curve. In this way, the add-arm design will show more powerful than the drop-arm design. At the same time, if several doses have similar response, the selection probabilities will be similar among doses and lower doses have a good chance to select. This is a desirable feature since higher doses are often associated with a higher cost or lower tolerability, and/or inconvenience.

Chang and Wang (2014) pointed out that the doses (arms) can be virtual doses, e.g., different drug combinations or different dose-schedule combinations. To increase power of the add-arm design, we can rearrange the dose (arm) sequence so that the most responsive arms are placed at or near the middle of the response curve. Such an arrangement is based on prior information, but mistakes can happen when the responses among the arms are similar, i.e., the arranged the arm (dose) sequence may not be unimodal. For this reason, comparisons of the designs are conservatively (unflavored to the add-arm design) based on the average power over all the response curves for the add-arm design to the power of the drop-loser design (Table 8.6).

8.5 Summary

We have studied the effective add-arm adaptive designs. Under unimodal responses (including linear and umbrella responses), the three-stage add-arm design is usually more powerful than the 2-stage drop-arm design mainly because the former takes the advantage of the knowledge of unimodality of responses. If the response is not unimodal, we can use that prior knowledge to rearrange the dose sequence so that it becomes a unimodal response.

In the add-arm design, all arms are usually selected with equal chance when all arms have the same expected response, but the probability of rejection is different even when all arms are equally effective. This feature allows us to effectively use the prior information to place more effective treatments in the middle at the first stage to increase the power.

In an add-arm design, dose levels don't have to be equally placed or based on the dose amount. The arms can be virtual dose levels or combinations of different drugs. Furthermore, the number of arms and the actual dose levels do not have to be prespecified, but instead, can be decided after the interim analyses.

As mentioned earlier, the constant c_R is usually so chosen to ensure the equal selection probability for a flat response curve. However, this requirement can be relaxed (slightly) if we want to have certain α spending among the arms to boost the correct selection probability and power if there is good information about dose-response curve availability. We further noticed that the stopping boundary c_α and α spending can be adjusted by modifying the c_R (slightly) and the information time τ.

The distribution of the final test statistic for the drop-arm design appears to be normal under H_G and H_a, whereas the distribution of the test statistic of the add-arm design appears to be normal under H_G and skewed under H_a.

Sample size can be reestimated at the interim analyses, but the distributions of test statistics and stopping boundaries will be different. The stopping boundary and power can be obtained using computer simulations.

We have assumed that a bigger response in the endpoint is better in previous discussions. For an endpoint for which a smaller value is better, we can change the sign of the variable or use other variable transform methods. When a smaller response rate is better, we can change the proportion of responses to the proportion of nonresponders as the endpoint, but keep the interpretation unchanged.

Chapter 9

Biomarker-Adaptive Design

9.1 Taxonomy

Biomarkers, as compared to a true (primary) endpoint such as survival, can often be measured earlier, easier, and more frequently and are less subject to competing risks, and less confounded. The utilization of biomarkers will lead to a better target population with a larger effect size, a smaller sample-size required, and faster decision-making. With the advancement of proteomic, genomic and genetic technologies, personalized medicine with the right drug for the right patient becomes possible.

Conley and Taube (2004) described the future of biomarker/genomic markers in cancer therapy: "The elucidation of the human genome and fifty years of biological studies have laid the groundwork for a more informed method for treating cancer with the prospect of realizing improved survival. Advanced in knowledge about the molecular abnormalities, signaling pathways influence the local tissue milieu and the relevance of genetic polymorphism offer hope of designing effective therapies tailored for a given cancer in particular individual, as well as the possibility of avoiding unnecessary toxicity."

Wang, Hung, and O'Neill (2006) from the FDA have pointed out: "Generally, when the primary clinical efficacy outcome in a phase III trial requires much longer time to observe, a surrogate endpoint thought to be strongly associated with the clinical endpoint may be chosen as the primary efficacy variable in phase II trials. The results of the phase II studies then provide an estimated effect size on the surrogate endpoint, which is supposedly able to help size the phase III trial for the primary clinical efficacy endpoint, where often it is thought to have a smaller effect size."

What exactly is a biomarker? A National Institutes of Health Workshop (Biomarkers Definition Working Group, 2001) gave the following definitions: *Biomarker* is a characteristic that is objectively measured and evaluated as an indicator of normal biologic processes, pathogenic processes, or pharmacological responses to a therapeutic intervention. *Clinical endpoint* (or outcome) is a characteristic or variable that reflects how a patient feels or functions, or how long a patient survives. *Surrogate endpoint* is a biomarker intended to substitute for a clinical endpoint. Biomarkers can also be classified as classifier, prognostic, and predictive biomarkers, but they are not mutually exclusive.

A classifier biomarker is a marker, e.g., a DNA marker, which usually does not change over the course of study. A classifier biomarker can be used to select the most appropriate target population or even for personalized treatment. For example, a study drug is expected to have effects on a population with a biomarker, which is only 20% of the overall patient population. Because the sponsor suspects that the drug may not work for the overall patient population, it may be efficient and ethical to run a trial only for the subpopulations with the biomarker rather than the general patient population. On the other hand, some biomarkers such as RNA markers are expected to change over the course of the study. This type of marker can be either a prognostic or predictive marker.

A prognostic biomarker informs the clinical outcomes, independent of treatment. It provides information about natural course of the disease in individuals with or without treatment under study. A prognostic marker does not inform the effect of the treatment. For example, Non-Small Cell Lung Cancer (NSCLC) patients receiving either EGFR inhibitors or chemotherapy have better outcomes with a mutation than without a mutation. Prognostic markers can be used to separate good and poor prognosis patients at the time of diagnosis. If expression of the marker clearly separates patients with an excellent prognosis from those with a poor prognosis, then the marker can be used to aid the decision about how aggressive the therapy needs to be. The poor prognosis patients might be considered for clinical trials of novel therapies that will, hopefully, be more effective (Conley and Taube, 2004). Prognostic markers may also inform the possible mechanisms responsible for the poor prognosis, thus leading to the identification of new targets for treatment and new effective therapeutics.

A predictive biomarker informs the treatment effect on the clinical endpoint. A predictive marker can be population-specific: a marker can be predictive for population A but not population B. A predictive biomarker, as compared to true endpoints like survival, can often be measured earlier, easier, and more frequently and is less subject to competing risks. For example, in a trial of a cholesterol-lowering drug, the ideal endpoint may be death or development of coronary artery disease (CAD). However, such a study usually requires thousands of patients and many years to conduct. Therefore, it is desirable to have a biomarker, such as a reduction in post-treatment cholesterol, if it predicts the reductions in the incidence of CAD.

In this chapter, we will discuss biomarker-enrichment design and biomarker-informed adaptive design.

Table 9.1: Response Rate and Sample-Size Required

	Population	RR_+	RR_-	Sample-size
Biomarker (+)	10M	50%	25%	160*
Biomarker (-)	40M	30%	25%	
Total	50M	34%	25%	1800

Note: *800 subjects screened. Power = 80%.

9.2 Biomarker-Enrichment Design

As mentioned earlier, a drug might have different effects in different patient populations. A hypothetical case is presented in Table 9.1, where RR_+ and RR_- are the response rates for biomarker-positive and biomarker-negative populations, respectively. In the example, there is a treatment effect of 25% in the 10 million patient population with the biomarker, but only 9% in the 50 million general patient populations. The sponsor faces the dilemma of whether to target the general patient population or use biomarkers to select a smaller set of patients that are expected to have a bigger response to the drug.

There are several challenges: (1) The estimated effect size for each subpopulation at the design stage is often very inaccurate; (2) a cost is associated with screening patients for the biomarker; (3) the test for detecting the biomarker often requires a high sensitivity and specificity, and the screening tool may not be available at the time of the clinical trial; and (4) screening patients for the biomarker may cause a burden and impact patient recruitment. These factors must be considered in the design.

Suppose we decide to run a trial on population with a biomarker. It is interesting to study how the screening testing will impact the expected utility. The size of the target patient size N with biomarker (+) can be expressed as

$$N = N_+ S_e + N_-(1 - S_p),   (9.1)$$

where N_+ and N_- are the sizes of patient populations with and without the biomarker, respectively; S_e is the sensitivity of the screening test, i.e., the probability of correctly identifying the biomarker among patients with the biomarker; and S_p is the specificity of the screening test, which is defined as the probability of correctly identifying biomarker-negative among patients without biomarkers. The average treatment effect for diagnostic biomarker (+) patients is

$$\delta = \frac{\delta_+ N_+ S_e + \delta_- N_-(1 - S_p)}{N}.   (9.2)$$

When the specificity increases, the target population decreases, but the average treatment effect in the target population increases because misdiagnosis of biomarker-negative as positive will reduce the average treatment effect.

Denote treatment difference between the test and control groups by δ_+, δ_-, and δ, for biomarker-positive, biomarker-negative, and overall patient populations, respectively. The null hypotheses are

$$\begin{cases} H_{01} : \delta_+ = 0 \text{ for biomarker-positive subpopulation,} \\ H_{02} : \delta_- = 0 \text{ for biomarker-negative subpopulation,} \\ H_0 : \delta = 0 \quad \text{for overall population.} \end{cases} \tag{9.3}$$

Without loss of generality, assume that the first n patients have the biomarker among N patients. We choose the test statistic for the trial as

$$T = \max\left(Z, Z_+\right). \tag{9.4}$$

It can be shown that the correlation coefficient between Z and Z_+ is

$$\rho = \sqrt{\frac{n}{N}}. \tag{9.5}$$

The distribution of T in (9.4) is given by Nadarajah and Kotz (2008).

Alternatively we can choose equal rejection boundary $z_{2,1-\alpha}$ or different stopping boundaries (c_1 and c_2) for the two correlated tests. Thus, the rejection boundary can be determined by

$$\Pr\left(T \geq z_{2,1-\alpha}|H_0\right) = \alpha, \tag{9.6}$$

where $z_{2,1-\alpha}$ is the bivariate normal $100(1-\alpha)$-equipercentage point under H_0.

The power can be calculated using

$$Power = \Pr\left(T \geq z_{2,1-\alpha}|H_a\right). \tag{9.7}$$

The numerical integration or simulations can be performed to evaluate $z_{2,1-\alpha}$ and the power.

Note that the test statistic for the overall population can be defined as

$$Z = w_1 Z_+ + w_2 Z_-, \tag{9.8}$$

where w_1 and w_2 are constants satisfying $w_1^2 + w_2^2 = 1$. In such a case, the correlation coefficient between Z and Z_+ is $\rho = w_1$. When the fixed weight is used we can do SSR at the interim analysis without inflating the type-I error.

To determine the critical point Z_c for rejecting the null at α level, run the simulations under the null condition for various Z_c until $\Pr\left(T > Z_c\right) \approx \alpha$. To determine the power, run the simulations under the alternative condition; the power is given by $\Pr\left(T > Z_c\right)$ or the percentage of the outcomes with $T > Z_c$.

We can also conduct an interim analysis and decide the target population at that time.

Table 9.2: Simulation Results of Two-Stage Design

Case	AveN	Power	pPower	oPower
H_o (Design 1)	700	0.025	0.013	0.013
H_a (Design 1)	672	0.09	0.59	0.31
H_o (Design 2)	550	0.025	0.01	0.02
H_a (Design 2)	564	0.09	0.55	0.35

Example 9.1: Biomarker-Enrichment Design

Suppose in an active-control two-group trial, the estimated treatment difference is 0.2 for the biomarker-positive population (BPP) and 0.05 for the biomarker-negative population (BNP) with a common standard deviation of $\sigma = 1.2$. Using R function (9.1), we can generate the operating characteristics under the global null hypothesis $H_0 : u_{0p} = 0 \cap u_{0n} = 0$, the alternative hypothesis $H_a : u_{0p} = 0.2 \cap u_{0n} = 0.05$ (see Table 9.2). We simulate the trials with two different sample size ratios, but both targeted 90% power and simulation results are presented in Table 9.2 and the typical R code for the simulation is presented in the following:

```
# Simulation of Global H0 Design 1 (Nn1=Nn2=200)
BiomarkerEnrichmentDesign(nSims=1000000,mup=0,    mun=0,    sigma=1.2,
Np1=200, Np2=200, Nn1=200, Nn2=200, c_alpha = 2.13)
# Simulation of Ha: Design 1 (Nn1=Nn2=200)
BiomarkerEnrichmentDesign(nSims=100000,mup=0.2,    mun=0.05,    sigma=1.2,
Np1=200, Np2=200, Nn1=200, Nn2=200, c_alpha = 2.13)
 # Simulation of Global H0 Design 2 (Nn1=Nn2=105)
                                      BiomarkerEnrichmentDe-
sign(nSims=1000000,mup=0, mun=0, sigma=1.2, Np1=210, Np2=210, Nn1=105,
Nn2=105, c_alpha = 2.39)
 # Simulation of H: Design 2 (Nn1=Nn2=105)
 BiomarkerEnrichmentDesign(nSims=100000,mup=0.2,    mun=0.05,    sigma=1.2,
Np1=210, Np2=210, Nn1=105, Nn2=105, c_alpha = 2.39)
```

9.3 Biomarker-Informed Adaptive Design

9.3.1 *Single-Level Model*

We have discussed the pick-the-winner designs where the same endpoint is used for both the interim and final analyses of the study. However, the benefits of such a design or method could be limited if it takes very long to obtain the primary endpoint measurements at the interim. For example, in oncology trials, it usually takes 12–24 months to observe overall survival: the most commonly used and preferred regulatory primary endpoint. The long time needed to reach the interim analyses can present potential operational challenges and may delay bringing a drug to the market.

Considerable interest has been drawn toward the short-term endpoint ("biomarker") informed adaptive seamless phase-II/III designs (Todd and Stallard, 2005; Shun et al., 2008; Stallard, 2010; Jenkins et al., 2010; Wang and Chang, 2014). These designs incorporate biomarker information at the interim stages of the study. The decision(s) on interim adaptation can be made based upon the biomarker only or on the available joint information of the biomarker and the primary endpoint. Biomarker-informed adaptive designs can be helpful for the development of personalized medicine, if the biomarker used at the interim is a good indicator of the primary endpoint.

The conventional one-level correlation model used for describing the relationship of the two endpoints in a biomarker-informed adaptive design considers only the individual level correlation (ρ). If the one-level correlation model is used in statistical simulations for biomarker-informed designs, the means of the two endpoints have to be specified based on the historical knowledge (as shown in Li et al., 2009).

$$\begin{pmatrix} Y_j \\ X_j \end{pmatrix} \sim N \left(\begin{pmatrix} \mu_{yj} \\ \mu_{xj} \end{pmatrix}, \begin{pmatrix} \sigma_y^2 & \rho\sigma_y\sigma_x \\ \rho\sigma_x\sigma_y & \sigma_x^2 \end{pmatrix} \right) \tag{9.9}$$

In this way, there would not be much difference in power among different values of correlation coefficient ρ between the biomarker and the primary endpoint. Friede et al. (2011) pointed out that the effect of the individual level correlation ρ between the endpoints on power is small if the means of the biomarker in treatment groups are fixed. The simulation results (Table 9.3) are consistent with the previous findings, where the interim sample size is 72, and the final sample size is 216.

We can see from Table 9.3 that if the conventional one-level correlation approach is used, when the correlation between the biomarker and the primary endpoint increases from 0.3 to 0.8, the simulated power of two-stage winner design changes from 96.48% to 97.37%. It is only slightly different. This

Table 9.3:Power of Winner Design with One-Level Correlation

ρ	Censoring Rate	Sample Size	Power	Power*
0.3	0.2	216	96.5%	66.7%
0.5	0.2	216	96.1%	66.3%
0.8	0.2	216	97.4%	67.7%

Power* = probability of rejection for the most arms.

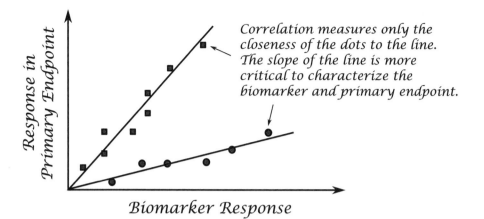

Figure 9.1: Relationships between Biomarker and Primary Endpoint

finding violates the presumption that the biomarker-informed design should have a better performance when the interim endpoint has a stronger correlation with the final endpoint.

Figure 9.1 illustrates different cases where the individual level correlation ρ between the biomarker and the primary endpoint is the same. Two different biomarkers (A and B) are described in the figure, both of which are correlated with the primary endpoint with correlation coefficient $\rho = 0.9$. Consider two designs, one uses biomarker A and the other uses biomarker B. Since only ρ is used in the conventional winner design, the two designs with the two different markers will give the same result. In fact, however, the knowledge about slope between the primary endpoint and biomarker is critical because by knowing the slope, we can know how much increase in biomarker in the interim means how much increase in the primary endpoint so that we can make wise decisions at the interim analysis. Therefore, it's not sufficient to describe the relationship between the biomarker and the primary endpoint by only considering the individual level correlation ρ. The uncertainties of μ_{yj}, μ_{yj}, or the slope, which is the rate of change of the primary endpoint with respect to the change in the biomarker, should also be incorporated in the trial design. The conventional one-level correlation model does not incorporate the variability of the slope caused by the uncertainty of historical data, which might easily lead to misestimated power.

If we can measure both responses in the biomarker and primary endpoint at the interim analysis, we can update the model (9.9). It might turn out that not only the ρ but all the parameters are very different. The problem is that we use biomarkers at interim analysis instead of the primary endpoint because we don't have enough observations on the primary endpoint at the interim. For the same reason, we cannot reliably update the model at the interim analysis.

9.3.2 *Hierarchical Model*

Instead of considering the parameters μ_{yj} and μ_{xj} the fixed parameters, we can naturally use the hierarchical (multilevel) model (MEM); that is, μ_{yj} and μ_{xj} follow a distribution:

$$
\begin{pmatrix} \mu_{yj} \\ \mu_{xj} \end{pmatrix} \sim N\left(\begin{pmatrix} \mu_{0yj} \\ \mu_{0xj} \end{pmatrix}, \begin{pmatrix} \sigma_{\mu_y}^2 & \rho_\mu \sigma_{\mu_y} \sigma_{\mu_x} \\ \rho_\mu \sigma_{\mu_x} \sigma_{\mu_y} & \sigma_{\mu_x}^2 \end{pmatrix} \right), \tag{9.10}
$$

where $i =$ treatment group and ρ and ρ_μ are the common correlations between individual and mean levels, respectively.

We can rewrite the distribution of $\begin{pmatrix} Y_j \\ X_j \end{pmatrix}$ in terms of the parameters in the parent model (9.10) by multiplying the pdfs (9.9) and (9.10), and integrating $\begin{pmatrix} \mu_{yj} \\ \mu_{xj} \end{pmatrix}$ out, which gives

$$
\begin{pmatrix} Y_j \\ X_j \end{pmatrix} \sim N\left(\begin{pmatrix} \mu_{0yj} \\ \mu_{0xj} \end{pmatrix}, \begin{pmatrix} \sigma_{\mu_y}^2 + \sigma_y^2 & \rho_\mu \sigma_{\mu_y} \sigma_{\mu_x} + \rho \sigma_y \sigma_x \\ \rho_\mu \sigma_{\mu_y} \sigma_{\mu_x} + \rho \sigma_y \sigma_x & \sigma_{\mu_x}^2 + \sigma_x^2. \end{pmatrix} \right) \tag{9.11}
$$

Note that all model parameters can be reassessed as the clinical trial data accumulated at each interim analysis using MLE or Bayesian posterior distribution.

Let's study this model and discuss how to implement this model into adaptive design. The implementation of biomarker-informed adaptive design with the hierarchical model is straightforward: (1) draw a sample $\begin{pmatrix} \mu_{yj} \\ \mu_{xj} \end{pmatrix}$ based on the distribution (9.10); (2) for each sample $\begin{pmatrix} \mu_{yj} \\ \mu_{xj} \end{pmatrix}$, draw N_1 samples of $\begin{pmatrix} Y_j \\ X_j \end{pmatrix}$ from (9.9) for the interim analysis based on biomarker X and determine the winner based on the best response in X; (3) draw additional $N_2 = N - N_1$ samples of the primary endpoint Y from the normal distribution $N\left(\mu_{yw}, \sigma_y^2\right)$ in the winner arm w and N samples of Y from $N\left(\mu_0, \sigma_0^2\right)$ for the placebo; and (4) test the hypothesis based on the primary endpoint Y at the final analysis, which will be based on data of the winner arm from the two stages and all the data of Y from placebo. The R-function for the biomarker-informed design with the hierarchical model is provided in Appendix B.

Table 9.4: Biomarker-Informed Design with MEM (ρ and σ Effects)

σ_μ	ρ_μ	σ	ρ	Power	Selection Probability
0.2	0	4	0.2	0.83	0.93, 0.06, 0.01
0.2	0.8	4	0.2	0.84	0.93, 0.06, 0.01
0.2	0	4	0.8	0.85	0.94, 0.06, 0.01
0.2	0.8	4	0.8	0.88	0.95, 0.05, 0.01
2	0.8	4	0.8	0.77	0.53, 0.28, 0.19
2	0.8	3	0.8	0.80	0.52, 0.28, 0.20

$\sigma_x = \sigma_y = \sigma$, $N_1 = 100$, $N = 300$.

For the purpose of simulation, we consider a placebo and three active arms with responses in the primary endpoints 0, 1, 0.5, and 0.2, respectively. The responses in the biomarker are 2, 1, and 0.5 for the three active arms, respectively. We don't need the biomarker response in the placebo arm.

We first try different critical values under the null hypothesis until the simulated power is equal to $\alpha = 0.025$. As a result, we obtain the critical value $= 2.772$. We then use this critical value to obtain power under the alternative hypothesis using simulations. The results are summarized in Table 9.4. We can see that even μ_{0yj} does not change; its variability σ_{μ_y} will impact the power significantly. When σ_{μ_y} is larger the power is less sensitive to the change of σ_y.

In the two-level relationship model, we study the effect of σ_r^2 on the power (Table 9.4). Similarly, for the hierarchical model we want to know how the changes of means from u_{xj} to cu_{xj} (c is a constant) will impact the power. We can see from the simulation results (Table 9.5) that the relationship between the primary endpoint means u_{yj} and biomarker means u_{xj} (see Figure 9.1) has a significant effect on the power.

Table 9.5: Biomarker-Informed Design with MEM (μ Effect)

u_{x1}	u_{x2}	u_{x3}	Power	Selection Probability
0.2	0.1	0.05	0.69	0.35, 0.33, 0.32
2	1	0.5	0.80	0.52, 0.28, 0.20
10	5	2.5	0.97	0.95, 0.05, 0.00
0.5	1	2	0.54	0.21, 0.28, 0.52
-2	-1	-0.5	0.57	0.18, 0.36, 0.46

$\sigma_x = \sigma_y = \sigma = 3$, $\sigma_{\mu y} = \sigma_{\mu x} = 2$, $\rho_\mu = \rho = 0.8$, $N_1 = 100$, $N = 300$.

Here are the codes to invoke the simulations:

```
## Determine critical value Zalpha for alpha (power) =0.025 ##
u0y=c(0,0,0); u0x=c(0,0,0)
powerBInfo(uCtl=0, u0y, u0x, rhou=1, suy=0, sux=0 ,rho=1, sy=4, sx=4, Zal-
pha=2.772, N1=100, N=300, nArms=3, nSims=100000)
## Power simulation ##
u0y=c(1,0.5,0.2)
u0x=c(2,1,0.5)
powerBInfo(uCtl=0, u0y, u0x, rhou=0.2, suy=0.2, sux=0.2 ,rho=0.2, sy=4, sx=4,
Zalpha=2.772, N1=100, N=300, nArms=3, nSims=5000)
```

9.4 Summary

Biomarker-informed adaptive design can shorten the time of drug development to bring the right drug to the right patient earlier, by incorporating a correlated short-term endpoint at the interim stages. Simulations should be performed before conducting such a clinical trial to understand the operating characteristics of the trial design. The conventional one-level correlation model used in simulations for the biomarker-informed adaptive designs might be inappropriate when the relationship between the biomarker and the primary endpoint is not well known. This model only considers the individual level correlation between the interim and final endpoint of the design. Uncertainty of the mean level relationship between the two endpoints is not considered. Hence, the simulation results of a biomarker-informed adaptive design using the conventional one-level model can easily misestimate the power.

The hierarchical model is an alternative way to effectively deal with biomarker utilization in clinical trials. We discussed how to use simulation to determine the critical value and how different parameters will affect the power and sample size. Such simulation studies should be conducted to decide whether the biomarker-informed design is better than the classical design or not.

Chapter 10

Response-Adaptive Randomization

10.1 Basic Response-Adaptive Randomizations

Response-adaptive randomization or allocation is a randomization technique in which the allocation of patients to treatment groups is based on the responses (outcomes) of the previous patients. The main purpose is to provide a better chance of randomizing the patients to a superior treatment group based on the knowledge about the treatment effect at the time of randomization. As a result, response-adaptive randomization takes ethical concerns into consideration. In the response-adaptive randomization, the response have not to be on the primary endpoint of the trial; instead, the randomization can be based on the response of a biomarker.

Perhaps the most commonly used response-adaptive randomization is the so-called randomized play-the-winner (RPW) model. RPW is a simple probabilistic model used to sequentially randomize subjects in a clinical trial (Wei and Durham, 1978; Coad and Rosenberger, 1999). The RPW model is useful for clinical trials comparing two treatments with binary outcomes. In the RPW model, it is assumed that the previous subject's outcome will be available before the next patient is randomized. At the start of the clinical trial, an urn contains a_0 balls representing treatment A and b_0 balls representing treatment B, where a_0 and b_0 are positive integers. We denote these balls as either type A or type B balls. When a subject is recruited, a ball is drawn and replaced. If it is a type A ball, the subject receives treatment A; if it is a type B ball, the subject receives treatment B. When a subject's outcome is available, the urn is updated as follows: A success on treatment A (B) or a failure on treatment B (A) will generate an additional a_1 (b_1) type-B balls in the urn. In this way, the urn builds up more balls representing the more successful treatment (Figure 10.1).

Example 10.1: Randomized Play-the-Winner Design

Suppose we are designing an oncology clinical study with tumor response as the primary endpoint. The response rate is estimated to be 0.3 in the

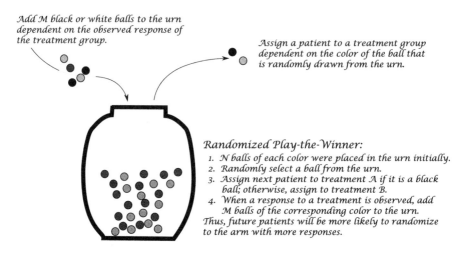

Figure 10.1:   Randomized Play-the-Winner

control group and 0.5 in the test group. The response rate is 0.4 in both groups under the null condition. We want to design the trial with about 80% power at a one-sided α of 0.025.

We will compare the simulation results for three different designs: (1) a classic design with a fixed sample size; (2) a group sequential design with 5 analyses, in which at each interim analysis the randomization is randomized based on the observed responses; and (3) a fully sequential design, in which the randomization is modified after each observation. The first step in the simulation is to determine the stopping boundary for each of the designs. This is because the adaptive randomization will change the distribution of the final test statistic and $zc = 1.96$ as the critical point for rejecting the null hypothesis for the classic design is not applicable to the adaptive randomization design anymore. The R code invoking the R function for the simulation is given below:

```
RPWBinary(nSims=10000, Zc=2.01, nSbjs=200, nAnlys=1, RR1=0.4, RR2=0.4,
a0=1, b0=1,a1=0, b1=0, nMin=1)
RPWBinary(nSims=1000, Zc=2.01, nSbjs=200, nAnlys=1, RR1=0.3, RR2=0.5,
a0=1, b0=1,a1=0, b1=0, nMin=1)
RPWBinary(nSims=10000, Zc=2.035, nSbjs=200, nAnlys=5, RR1=0.4, RR2=0.4,
a0=2, b0=2,a1=1, b1=1, nMin=1)
RPWBinary(nSims=1000, Zc=2.035, nSbjs=200, nAnlys=5, RR1=0.3, RR2=0.5,
a0=2, b0=2,a1=1, b1=1, nMin=1)
RPWBinary(nSims=10000,    Zc=2.010,    nSbjs=200,    nAnlys=200,    RR1=0.4,
RR2=0.4, a0=1, b0=1,a1=0, b1=0, nMin=1)
```

Table 10.1: Simulation Results from RPW

Design	nSbjs	aveP1	aveP2	Zc	Power
Classic design	200	0.300	0.500	2.010	0.81
5-Analysis GSD	200	0.292	0.498	2.050	0.80
Fully sequential	200	0.294	0.498	2.010	0.81

Note: 100,000 Simulation runs.

RPWBinary(nSims=1000, Zc=2.010, nSbjs=200, nAnlys=200, RR1=0.3, RR2=0.5, a0=1, b0=1,a1=0, b1=0, nMin=1)

The simulation results are summarized in Table 10.1, where aveP1 and aveP2 are the average proportion for the groups one and two, respectively. We can see that there is a slight loss in power using the group sequential design from the classic design, but there is virtually no difference between fully sequential design and the group sequential design.

Similarly we can study the characteristics of different urns by, for example, setting the parameters: $a_0 = 2$, $b_0 = 2$, $a_1 = 1$, $b_1 = 1$ for RPW (2,2,1,1). We left this for readers to practice.

10.2 Generalized Response-Adaptive Randomization

For other types of endpoints, we suggest the following allocation probability model:

$$\Pr(trt = i) = f(\hat{\mathbf{u}}), \qquad (10.1)$$

where $\Pr(trt = i)$ is the probability of allocating the patient to the ith group and the observed response vector $\hat{\mathbf{u}} = \{u_1, \ldots, u_M\}$.

We further suggest a specific function for f, i.e.,

$$\Pr(trt = i) \propto a_{0i} + b\,\hat{u}_i^m, \qquad (10.2)$$

where $\hat{u}_i$ = the observed proportion, mean, number of events, or categorical score, and a_{0i} and b are constants.

Example 10.2: Adaptive Randomization with Normal Endpoint

The objective of this trial in asthma patients is to confirm sustained treatment effect, measured as FEV1 change from baseline to 1 year of treatment. Initially, patients are equally randomized to four doses of the new compound and a placebo. Based on early studies, the estimated FEV1 change at week 4 are 6%, 12%, 13%, 14%, and 15% (with pooled standard deviation 18%) for the placebo, dose levels 1, 2, 3, and 4, respectively.

Using the following R code, we can determine that the rejection region is $(2.01, +\infty)$ for 375 subjects and $(1.995, +\infty)$ for 285 subjects. The power is 84% with a total of 375 subjects and 73% with 285 subjects, while the pick-the-winner design in Chapter 7 provides 85% with total sample size 289.

Here is the R code showing you how to to invoke the R function for the simulations:

```
# Simulation of H0
a0=rep(1,5); us=rep(0.06,5); s=rep(.18,5)
RARNorm(nSims=10000, nPts=375, nArms=5, b=1, m=1, CrtMax=2.01)
# Simulation of Ha
a0=rep(1,5); us=c(0.06, 0.12, 0.13, 0.14, 0.15); s=rep(.18,5)
RARNorm(nSims=10000, nPts=375, nArms=5, b=1, m=1, CrtMax=2.01)
```

It is interesting to know that many adaptive designs can be viewed as response-adaptive randomization design. We are going to illustrate this with the classical group sequential design and the drop-loser design.

For a two-arm group sequential design, the treatment allocation probability to the ith arm at the kth stage is given by

$$\Pr(trt = i; k) = \frac{H(p_k - \alpha_k) + H(\beta_k - p_k)}{2} - \frac{1}{2}, \tag{10.3}$$

where $i = 1, 2$, α_k and β_k are the stopping boundaries at the kth stage and the step-function is defined as

$$H(x) = \begin{cases} 1, & \text{if } x > 0 \\ 0 & \text{if } x \le 0 \end{cases}. \tag{10.4}$$

From (10.3), we can see that if $p_k \le \alpha_k$ (or $p_k \ge \beta_k$), the allocation probability $\Pr(trt = i; k)$ is zero, meaning the trial will stop for efficacy (or futility). If $\alpha_k < p_k < \beta_k$, the allocation probability $\Pr(trt = i; k)$ is 1/2, meaning the patients will be assigned to the two treatment groups with an equal probability. For drop-loser designs, if the dropping criterion is based on the maximum difference among the observed treatment $\hat{u}_{max} - \hat{u}_{min}$ at the interim analysis, then the treatment allocation probability to the ith arm at interim analysis is given by

$$\Pr(trt = i) = \frac{H(\hat{u}_i - \hat{u}_{max} + \delta_{NI})}{\sum_{i=1}^{M} H(\hat{u}_i - \hat{u}_{max} + \delta_{NI})}, \tag{10.5}$$

where $\hat{u}_i$ is the observed response in the ith arm, and δ_{NI} is the noninferiority margin. $M =$ the total number of arms in the study.

10.3   Summary and Discussion

Response-adaptive randomization (RAR) was initially proposed to reduce the number of failures in a trial; however, the overall gain is sometimes limited in a two-group design because (1) power is lost as compared to the uniformly most powerful design, and (2) the reduction in number of failures can diminish due to significantly delayed responses. RAR may (although it is unlikely) delay patient enrollment because of the fact that patients enrolled later will have a better chance of being assigned to a better treatment group. If there is heterogeneity in patient enrollment over time (e.g., sicker patients tend to enroll earlier because they cannot wait for long), a bias will be introduced.

RAR may be useful in phase-II/III combination studies, where at the early stages, RAR is used to seamlessly select superior arms. In practice, group (rather than full) sequential response-adaptive randomization may be used, where the response data will be unblinded at several prescheduled times. Sequential parallel comparison design (SPCD) is a special response-adaptive design, which has practical applications, such as in psychiatry trials.

Chapter 11

Adaptive Dose-Escalation Trial

In this chapter, we will introduce two commonly used approaches for oncology dose-escalation trials: (1) the algorithm-based escalation rules, and (2) model-based approaches. The second approach can be a frequentist or Bayesian-based response-adaptive method and can be used in any dose-response trials.

11.1 Oncology Dose-Escalation Trial

For non-life-threatening diseases, since the expected drug toxicity is mild and can be controlled without harm, phase-I trials are usually conducted on healthy or normal volunteers. However, in life-threatening diseases such as cancer and AIDS, phase-I studies are conducted with a limited number of patients due to (1) the aggressiveness and possible harmfulness of cytotoxic treatments, (2) possible systemic treatment effects, and (3) the high interest in the new drug's efficacy in those patients directly.

Drug toxicity is considered as tolerable if the toxicity is manageable and reversible. The standardization of the level of drug toxicity is the Common Toxicity Criteria (CTC) developed by the United States National Cancer Institute (NCI). Any adverse event (AE) related to treatment of CTC category of grade 3 and higher is often considered a dose-limiting toxicity (DLT). The maximum tolerated dose (MTD) is defined as the maximum dose with a DLT rate that is no more frequent than a predetermined value.

11.1.1 *Dose Level Selection*

The initial dose given to the first patients in a phase-I study should be low enough to avoid severe toxicity. The commonly used starting dose is the dose at which 10% mortality (LD_{10}) occurs in mice. The subsequent dose levels are usually selected based on the following multiplicative set: $x_i = f_{i-1}x_{i-1}$ ($i = 1, 2, ...K$), where f_i is called the dose-escalation factor. The highest dose level should be selected such that it covers the biologically active dose, but remains lower than the toxic dose. A popular dose-escalation factor is called the Fibonacci sequence (2, 1.5, 1.67, 1.60, 1.63, 1.62, 1.62, ...) and modified Fibonacci sequence (2, 1.65, 1.52, 1.40, 1.33, 1.33, ...). Note that the latter is a monotonic sequence and hence more appropriate than the former.

11.1.2 *Traditional Escalation Rules*

There are usually 5 to 10 predetermined dose levels with modified Fibonacci sequence in a dose-escalation study. Patients are treated with the lowest dose first and then gradually escalated to higher doses if there is no major safety concern. The rules for dose escalation are predetermined. The commonly employed set of dose-escalation rules is the traditional escalation rules (TERs), also known as the "3+3" rule. The "3+3" rule says to enter three patients at a new dose level and enter another 3 patients when only one DLT is observed. The assessment of the six patients will be performed to determine whether the trial should be stopped at that level or to increase the dose. Basically, there are two types of the "3+3" rules, namely, TER and strict TER (or STER). TER does not allow dose deescalation, but STER does. The "3+3" TER and STER can be generalized to "$A + B$" TER and STER.

To introduce the $A + B$ escalation rule, let $A, B, C, D,$ and E be integers. The notation A/B indicates that there are A toxicity incidences out of B subjects and $>A/B$ means that there are more than A toxicity incidences out of B subjects. We assume that there are K predefined doses and let p_i be the probability of observing a DLT at dose level i for $1 \leq i \leq K$.

A+B Escalation without Dose Deescalation

The general $A + B$ designs without dose deescalation can be described as follows. Suppose that there are A patients at dose level i. If fewer than C/A patients have DLTs, then the dose is escalated to the next dose level $i + 1$. If more than D/A (where $D \geq C$) patients have DLTs, then the previous dose $i - 1$ will be considered the MTD. If no fewer than C/A but no more than D/A patients have DLTs, B more patients are treated at this dose level i. If no more than E (where $E \geq D$) of the total of $A + B$ patients experience DLTs, then the dose is escalated. If more than E of the total of $A + B$ patients have DLT, then the previous dose $i - 1$ will be considered the MTD. It can be seen that the traditional "3+3" design without dose deescalation is a special case of the general $A + B$ design with $A = B = 3$ and $C = D = E = 1$. Lin and Shih (2001) derived the closed forms of operating characteristics.

A+B Escalation with Dose Deescalation

Basically, the general $A + B$ design with dose deescalation is similar to the design without dose deescalation. However, it permits more patients to be treated at a lower dose (i.e., dose deescalation) when excessive DLT incidences occur at the current dose level. The dose deescalation occurs when more than D/A (where $D \geq C$) or more than $E/(A+B)$ patients have DLTs at dose level i. In this case, B more patients will be treated at dose level $i-1$, provided that only A patients have been previously treated at this prior dose. If more than A patients have already been treated previously, then dose $i-1$ is the MTD. The deescalation may continue to the next dose level $i-2$ and so on if necessary. The closed forms of operating characteristics are given by Lin and Shih (2001) as follows.

Aiming to increase in-trial patient safety without unnecessary increase in sample size, Lee and Fan (2012) proposed a two-dimensional search algorithm for dose-finding trials of two agents, which uses not only the frequency but also the source of dose-limiting toxicities to direct dose escalations and deescalations. In addition, when the doses of both agents are escalated simultaneously, a more conservative design replaces a default aggressive design to evaluate the resulting dose combination.

11.2 Continual Reassessment Method

The continual reassessment method (CRM) is a model approach, in which the parameters in the model for the response are continually updated based on the observed response data. CRM was initially proposed by O'Quigley (O'Quigley, et al., 1990; O'Quigley and Shen, 1996) for oncology dose-escalation trial. However, it can be extended to other types of trials (Chang and Chow, 2005).

11.2.1 *Reassessment of Parameter*

Probability Model for Dose-Response

Let x be the dose or dose level, and $p(x)$ be the probability of response or response rate. The commonly used model for dose-response is a logistic toxicity model (Figure 11.1).

$$P(x) = [1 + b\exp(-ax)]^{-1}, \qquad (11.1)$$

where b is usually a predetermined constant and a is a parameter to be updated based on observed data.

Likelihood Function

The next step is to construct the likelihood function. Given n observations with y_i $(i = 1, \ldots, n)$ associated with dose x_{m_i}, the likelihood function can be written as

$$f_n(\mathbf{r}\,|a) = \prod_{i=1}^{n} [p(x_{m_i})]^{r_i}\, [1 - p(x_{m_i})]^{1-r_i}, \qquad (11.2)$$

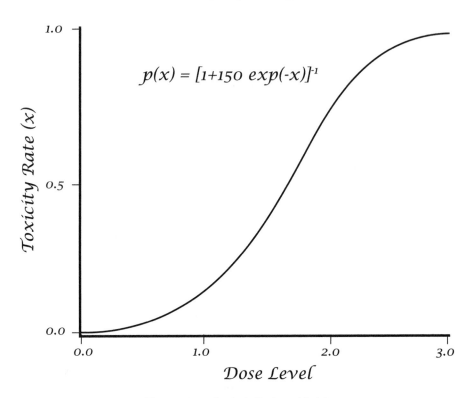

Figure 11.1:   Logistic Toxicity Model

where

$$r_i = \begin{cases} 1, & \text{if response observed for } x_{m_i} \\ 0, & \text{otherwise} \end{cases} . \tag{11.3}$$

Prior Distribution of Parameter

The Bayesian approach requires the specification of prior probability distribution of the unknown parameter a:

$$a \sim g_0(a), \tag{11.4}$$

where $g_0(a)$ is the prior probability distribution.

When very limited knowledge about the prior is available, non-informative prior can be used.

Reassessment of Parameter

The key is to estimate the parameter a in the response model (11.1). An initial assumption or a prior about the parameter is necessary in order to assign patients to the dose level based on the dose-toxicity relationship. This estimation of a is continually updated based on the cumulative response data observed from the trial thus far. The estimation method can be a Bayesian or frequentist approach. A Bayesian approach leads to the posterior distribution of a. For frequentist approaches, a maximum likelihood estimate or least square estimate can be used.

The posterior probability of parameter a can be obtained as follows

$$g_n(a|\mathbf{r}) = \frac{f_n(\mathbf{r}|a)g_0(a)}{\int f_n(\mathbf{r}|a)g_0(a)\,da} \tag{11.5}$$

or

$$g_n(a|\mathbf{r}) = \frac{[p_n(a)]^{r_n}[1-p_n(a)]^{1-r_n}g_{n-1}(a)}{\int [p_n(a)]^{r_n}[1-p_n(a)]^{1-r_n}g_{n-1}(a)\,da}, \tag{11.6}$$

where $p_n(a) = p(x_{m_n})$ is the response rate at the dose level, at which the nth patient is treated.

11.2.2 *Assignment of Next Patient*

After having obtained $g_n(a|\mathbf{r})$, we can update the predictive probability using

$$P(x) = \int [1 + b\exp(-ax)]^{-1}g_n(a|\mathbf{r})\,da. \tag{11.7}$$

The updated dose-toxicity model is usually used to choose the dose level for the next patient. In other words, the next patient enrolled in the trial is assigned to the currently estimated MTD based on the predictive probability (11.7). Practically, this assignment is subject to safety constraints such as limited dose jump. Assignment of patients to the most updated MTD is intuitive. This way, a majority of the patients will be assigned to the dose levels near MTD, which allows for a more precise estimation of MTD with a minimal number of patients.

In practice, if is also not ethical to make a big dose jump. We usually implement a limitation on dose jump, e.g., a dose can only be escalated one dose level high at one time.

11.2.3 *Stopping Rule*

As soon as a certain number of patients (e.g., 6 patients) is recruited at a single dose level, the trial will stop. This is because, for example, when there are 6 patients at a dose level, it means that the model has predicted the MTD at the same dose level 6 times; thus it is reasonable to believe this dose level is the MTD. We don't want all dose levels to have 6 patients since it would not be an efficient design.

11.3   Alternative Form CRM

The CRM is often presented in an alternative form (e.g.,Yin and Yuan, 2011). In practice, we usually prespecify the doses of interest, instead of any dose. Let $(d_1, \ldots, d_K)$ be a set of dose and $(p_1, \ldots, p_K)$ be the corresponding prespecified probability, called the "skeleton," satisfying $p_1 < p_2, \ldots < p_K$. The dose-toxicity model of the CRM is assumed, instead of (11.1), to be

$$\Pr(\text{toxicity at } d_i) = \pi_i(a) = p_i^{\exp(a)}, i = 1, 2, \ldots, K, \qquad (11.8)$$

where a is an unknown parameter. Parabolic tangents or logistic structures can also be used to model the dose-toxicity curve.

Let D be the observed data: y_i out of n_i patients treated at dose level i have experienced the dose-limiting toxicity (DLT). Based on the binomial distribution, the likelihood function is

$$L(D|a) \propto \prod_{i=1}^{K} \left\{ p_i^{\exp(a)} \right\}^{y_i} \left(1 - p_i^{\exp(a)} \right)^{n_i - y_i}. \qquad (11.9)$$

Using Bayes' theorem, the posterior means of the toxicity probabilities at dose j can be computed by

$$\hat{\pi}_i = \frac{1}{\int L(D|a) g_0(a) \, da} \int p_i^{\exp(a)} L(D|a) g_0(a) \, da, \qquad (11.10)$$

where $g_0(a)$ is a prior distribution for a, for example, $a \sim N\left(0, \sigma^2\right)$.

11.4   Evaluation of Dose-Escalation Design

There are advantages and disadvantages with different dose-escalation schemes. For example, the traditional 3+3 escalation is easy to apply but the MTD estimation is usually biased, especially when there are many dose levels. The criteria for evaluation of escalation schemes are listed as follows: the number of DLTs, number of patients, number of patients dosed above MTD, accuracy, and precision.

Before a phase-I trial is initiated, the following design characteristics should be checked and defined in the study protocol: (1) starting dose, (2) dose levels, (3) prior information on the MTD, (4) toxicity model, (5) escalation rule, (6) stopping rule, and (7) rules for completion of the sample-size when stopping.

Example 11.1: Adaptive Dose-Finding for Prostate Cancer Trial

A trial is designed to establish the dose-toxicity relationship and identify MTD for a compound in patients with metastatic androgen independent

Table 11.1: Dose Levels and DLT Rates

Dose level i	1	2	3	4	5	6	7	8
Dose x	30	45	68	101	152	228	342	513
DLT rate	0.01	0.02	0.03	0.05	0.12	0.17	0.22	0.4

prostate cancer. Based on preclinical data, the estimated MTD is 230 mg/m^2. The modified Fibonacci sequence is chosen for the dose levels (in Table 11.1). There are 8 dose levels anticipated, but more dose levels can be added if necessary. The initial dose level is 30 mg/m^2, which is 1/10 of the minimal effective dose level (mg/m^2) for 10% deaths (MELD10) of the mouse after verification that no lethal and no life-threatening effects were seen in another species. The toxicity rate (DLT rate) at MTD is defined for this indication as 17%.

For logistic toxicity model, $p = \frac{1}{1+150\exp(-a\,i)}$ is used, where $i =$ dose level (we can also use actual dose) and the prior distribution for parameter a is flat over [0, 0.8]. For the skeleton toxicity model $p_i^{\exp(a)}$, the following skeleton is used: $p_i = (.01, .02, .04, .08, .16, .32, .4, .5)$ and a flat prior a over [-0.1, 2]. The R code invoking the CRM function is presented here:

```
#Logistic Model
g= c(1); doses = c(1)
RRo = c(0.01,0.02,0.03,0.05,0.12,0.17,0.22,0.4)
for (k in 1:100) {g[k]=1}; # Flat prior
for (i in 1:8) {doses[i]=i}
CRM(nSims=500, nPts=30, nLevels=8, b=150, aMin=0, aMax=3,
MTRate=0.17, ToxModel="Logist", nPtsForStop=6)
#Skeleton Model
g = c(1); doses = c(1)
RRo = c(0.01,0.02,0.03,0.05,0.12,0.17,0.22,0.4)
skeletonP=c(0.01,0.02,0.04,0.08,0.16,0.32,0.4,0.5)
for (k in 1:100) {g[k]=1}; # Flat prior
CRM(nSims=500, nPts=20, nLevels=8, aMin=-0.1, aMax=2,
MTRate=0.17, ToxModel="Skeleton", nPtsForStop=6)
```

The simulation results are presented in Table 11.2. In addition, the percent or the probabilities of selecting different dose levels as the MTD are also obtained from the simulations: for CRM logistic model they are 0, 0, 0, .0001, 0.4, 0.3446, 0.1159, and 0.1394 for dose 1 to dose 8, respectively. For CRM skeleton model, the selecting probabilities are 0, 0, 0, 0, 0.1379, 0.5305, 0.1776, and 0.154 for the 8 doses.

Note that the true MTD is dose level 6 (228 mg/m^2). The average predicted MTD (dose level) is 5.97 with TER. In contrast, the average MTD

Table 11.2: Adaptive Dose-Response Simulation Results

Method	Mean N	Mean DLTs	Mean MTD	SdMTD
TER	24.5	2.71	5.97	1.43
CRM (Logistic)	17.9	2.10	5.03	1.85
CRM (Skeleton)	14.3	2.28	6.20	0.92

for CRM with logistic toxicity model is dose level 5.03, lower than the target level. The average MTD for CRM with toxicity skeleton is level 6.20 and requires an average sample-size of 14.3 and a mean DLT of 2.28. From a precision point of view, even with a smaller sample-size, the standard deviation of MTD (SdMTD) is smaller for CRM (skeleton) than TER. However, we should be aware that the performance of CRM is dependent on the goodness of the model specification.

```
#Logistic Model
g= c(1); doses = c(1)
RRo = c(0.01,0.02,0.03,0.05,0.12,0.17,0.22,0.4)
for (k in 1:100) {g[k]=1}; # Flat prior
for (i in 1:8) {doses[i]=i}
CRM(nSims=500, nPts=30, nLevels=8, b=150, aMin=0, aMax=3,
MTRate=0.17, ToxModel="Logist", nPtsForStop=6)
#Skeleton Model
g = c(1); doses = c(1)
RRo = c(0.01,0.02,0.03,0.05,0.12,0.17,0.22,0.4)
skeletonP=c(0.01,0.02,0.04,0.08,0.16,0.32,0.4,0.5)
for (k in 1:100) {g[k]=1}; # Flat prior
CRM(nSims=500, nPts=20, nLevels=8, aMin=-0.1, aMax=2,
MTRate=0.17, ToxModel="Skeleton", nPtsForStop=6)
```

11.5 Summary and Discussion

We have studied the traditional algorithm-based and model-based approaches for dose-response trials. The efficiencies of the approaches are dependent on several aspects, such as the situation in which the next patient is enrolled before we have the response data from the previous patient. In this case, the efficacy of the TER and CRM may be reduced. There may also be a limit for dose escape, which may also reduce the efficiency of the CRM.

   In addition to $A + B$ escalation algorithms, many other algorithms have been proposed (Chevret, 2006 and Ting, 2006). For example, Shih and Lin

(2006) modified $A + B$ and derived closed form solutions for the modified algorithms. They were motivated by the following: (1) In a traditional $A + B$ design, the previous dose level is always declared the maximum tolerated dose (MTD), and the current dose has no chance at all of being declared the MTD; (2) the starting dose cannot necessarily be the lowest dose; and (3) the design may be a two-stage escalation design used to accelerate the escalation in the early part of the trial with one or two patients per dose level. However, the values from (1) and (2) are questionable because any dose can be the current or previous dose level, and just like dose jump, dosing the first patient at a higher dose level may put certain individuals at risk, even though the overall toxicity (e.g., number of DLTs) may be reduced.

CRM can be used with other monotonic or nonmonotonic models and can be combined with response-adaptive randomization or a drop-loser design (Chang and Chow, 2005).

Chapter 12

Deciding Which Adaptive Design to Use

When you design the very first adaptive trial, you want to know how to start; you may even wonder in the adaptive design would really be better than if classic design. What if I miss something or something goes wrong? Don't worry; this chapter we discuss the process and build your confidence in designing an adaptive trial.

The first step is to choose an appropriate type of adaptive design based on the trial objective(s). If it is a phase-III confirmatory trial, we may consider group sequential design or SSR design. Further, if the timing of the analyses or the number of analyses are expected to change due to practical reasons (e.g., the availability of DMC committee members or safety concerns about the need to add more interim analyses), we should choose GSD with error-spending approach; if the estimation of effect size is very unreliable, we should use SSR. Generally, the mixed method for SSR is recommended since it is usually more effective in bringing back the power when effect size is lower than expected. And the mixed method does not fully unblind the effect size to the sponsor and the general public, which is an attractive mechanism to protect the integrity of the adaptive trial. If dose (arm) to be considered is more than two (including the control arm) since, for example, we don't know exactly which dose (treatment regimens or combinations of drugs) is the best (or good enough), we should use an add-arm or drop-arm design. An add-arm design is usually statistically more efficient than a drop-arm design, but also adds a little more to the complexity of the trial design and conduct. We should perform the clinical trial simulations to further evaluate and compare the operating characteristics of different designs or designs with different parameters. If the trial is an early stage design for a progressive disease such as cancer, we can use dose-escalation design, in which the dose gradually increases to protect the patients' safety. If a screening test of a stable biomarker is available (and practical) and we expect the test drug may have different efficacy and/or safety profiles for patients with and without the biomarker, we can use a biomarker enrichment design, in which the interim analysis will be used for deciding which population should be the target. If the biomarker is expected to respond to the drug and it can be measured earlier at the interim analysis than the primary endpoint of the trial, then we can use a biomarker-informed adaptive design. The response-adaptive design can be based on the primary endpoint or the biomarker response if the former is not available at the time of randomization.

The next step is to determine whether a superiority, noninferiority, or equivalence trial is needed based on the primary trial objective and the regulatory requirement. The timing and number of interim analyses will be dependent on the safety requirement (some need more frequent safety monitoring), statistical efficiency (more interim analyses might reduce the sample size; need CTS to check), practicality (complexity of the trial conduct and associated time and cost). You may need to consider some special issues, such as paired data, missing data, etc. Conduct simulations to see which method (MSP, MINP, MPP) will give you the most efficient design. Conduct broad simulations with various design features/parameters and choose the most appropriate one based on the proposed evaluation matrix. Note that classical designs are often used as the basis for the comparisons of different trial designs. Finally, we need to consider the practical issues: How long will the trial take? Should we halt the trial when we perform the interim analysis? How fast can we do the interim analysis including the data cleaning? Will the recruitment speed and delayed response jeopardize the adaptive design? Who will perform the interim analysis and write the interim monitoring plan or DMC Charter? Does the regulatory agency agree on the noninferiority margin if a noninferiority adaptive trial? How will the randomization be done? Can IVRS (interactive voice response system) support the adaptive design? How will the drug be distributed to the clinic sites? How will the primary analysis for the adaptive trial data be done? See Figure 12.1: Adaptive Clinical Trial Flow Chart.

12.1 Determining the Objectives

The trial objectives are determined by the study team in the company. What a statistician can do is to prioritize the objectives based on the clinical and commercial objectives and optimize the trial design to increase the likelihood of success.

12.2 Determining Design Parameters

12.2.1 *Model Parameters*

First we determine the primary endpoint, a normal, binary, or survival endpoint; the timing when the endpoint should be measured; weather it is based

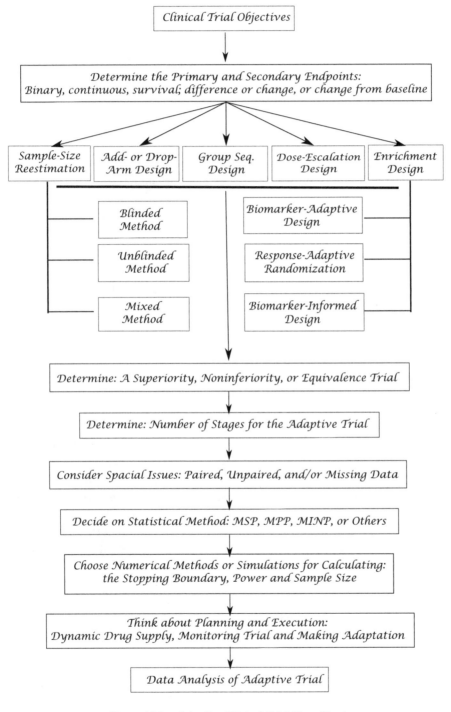

Figure 12.1:   Adaptive Clinical Trial Flow Chart

on the change from baseline or the raw measure at a postbaseline. After determining the endpoint, we need to estimate the expected value for the endpoint in each treatment group based on prior information, which might be an early clinical trial, a preclinical study, and/or published clinical trial results by other companies for the same class drug. The reliability of the historical data will affect your choice of the adaptive design.

12.2.2 *Determine the Thresholds for α and β*

For phase-III trials, the type-I error rate must be controlled at one-sided significance level $\alpha = 0.025$; for early phase trials, α can be flexible. A smaller α will reduce the false positive drug candidate entering late-phase trials, but at the same time increase the chance of eliminating the effective drug candidates from further studies, unless we increase the sample size to keep the type-II error rate β unchanged.

12.2.3 *Determine the Stopping Boundaries*

The most important factors (operation characteristics) for selecting a design with interim analyses are the expected sample size and maximum sample size. If you wish to reduce the expected cost, you might want to choose a design with minimum expected sample size; if you wish to reduce the maximum possible cost, you might want to consider a design with minimum total sample size. In any case, you should carefully compare all the stopping probabilities between different designs before determining an appropriate design. O'Brien-Fleming's boundary is very conservative in early rejecting the null hypothesis. The Pocock boundary applies a constant boundary on p-scale across different stages. Generally speaking, a large delta (e.g., 0.8) will lead to a design that spends type-I error more at earlier stages than later stages. To increase the probability of accepting the null hypothesis at earlier stages, a futility boundary can be used. If you don't want to accept the null hypothesis at interim analyses, you should choose a design with rejection to the null hypothesis only. On the other hand, if you don't want to reject the null hypothesis at interim analyses, you should choose a design with acceptance of the null hypothesis only. In general, if you expect the effect size of the treatment is less than what you have assumed and the cost is your main concern, you should use an aggressive futility boundary to give a larger stopping probability at the interim in case the drug is ineffective or less effective. On the other hand, if you worry that the effect size might be underestimated, you should design the trial with aggressive efficacy stopping boundary (Pocock-like rather than O'Brian-Fleming-like) to boost the probability early efficacy stopping in case the drug is very effective.

12.3   Evaluation Matrix of Adaptive Design

To choose an adaptive design among several options, we have to consider the trial objective, the cost, the duration of the study, the recruitment challenges, execution challenges, and how to get team and regulatory authority buy-in. We can consider the impact of failure and success of the trial using a utility function:

$$U = \int R_i(\boldsymbol{\theta})w_i f(\boldsymbol{\theta}) \, d\boldsymbol{\theta}, \tag{12.1}$$

where $\boldsymbol{\theta}$ is the design input parameter vector, R_i is outcome or result vector component or operating characteristics, w_i is the corresponding weight measuring the relative importance of R_i among all Rs, and $f(\boldsymbol{\theta})$ is the prior distribution of $\boldsymbol{\theta}$.

Practically, for the expected sample size we can simplify using an approximation:

$$\bar{N} = \Pr(H_0) N_0 + \Pr(H_s) N_s + \Pr(H_a) N_a. \tag{12.2}$$

For instance, if we believe $\Pr(H_0) = 0.2$, $\Pr(H_s) = 0.2$, and $\Pr(H_a) = 0.6$, then $\bar{N} = 0.2N_0 + 0.2N_s + 0.6N_a$, where the sample sizes N_0, N_s, and N_a are the three expected sample sizes under H_0, H_s, and H_a, respectively.

12.3.1   *Group Sequential Design*

Design input parameters: three (or more)treatment difference θ_1, θ_2, and θ_3 and the associate probabilities, $\Pr(H_0 : \theta_1)$, $\Pr(H_s : \theta_2)$, and $\Pr(H_a : \theta_3)$; number of analyses; timing of analyses; futility and efficacy stopping boundaries; error-spending function

Design outcome parameters (operating characteristics): the expected sample sizes under H_0, H_s, H_a, and their weighted average $\bar{N}$ by (12.2); the maximum sample size N_{max}; number of analyses; power, utility, safety management; complexity of the trial design and conduct

For the comparisons of different GSDs, we usually fix the power for different designs and compare the average sample size or utility. For example, suppose we select the following three designs for comparison: design 1: 2-stage GSD without futility stopping boundary, design 2: 3-stage GSD without futility stopping boundary, and design 3: 2-stage GSD with futility stopping boundary. We run the simulation using different input parameters for the three designs and tabulate the outputs in Table 12.1:

Table 12.1: Group Sequential Design Evaluation Matrix

Design	N̄	Nmax	Safety	Complexity	Power	Utility
1						
2						
3						

Table 12.2: Sample-Size Reestimation Evaluation Matrix

Design	N̄	Nmax	Safety	Complexity	Power	Utility

12.3.2   *Sample-Size Reestimation Design*

Design input parameters: treatment differences θ_1, θ_2, and θ_3 and the associate probabilities, $\Pr(H_0 : \theta_1)$, $\Pr(H_s : \theta_2)$, and $\Pr(H_a : \theta_3)$; number of analyses; timing of analyses; futility and efficacy stopping boundaries. The evaluation matrix is the sample as for GSDs (Table 12.2):

12.3.3   *Dose-Finding Trial (Add-Arm, Drop-Arm Design)*

When using a drop-arm design, we don't need to worry about the dose-response pattern, but we need to arrange the arms (doses) with our best knowledge into a unimodal response-curve.

Design input parameters: number of arms, total number of subjects, the treatment effect for each arm or dose response curve, timing of analyses, interim selection criteria, futility and efficacy stopping boundaries

Design outcome parameters (operating characteristics): distribution of selection probability, power, safety, operation complexity including duration of the study (Table 12.3):

12.3.4   *Response-Adaptive Randomization*

Design input parameters: total number of subjects, parameters of the randomization urn (a0, b0, a1, b1), treatment effect for each arm. The evaluation matrix is presented in Table 12.4:

Table 12.3: Add-Arm, Drop-Arm Evaluation Matrix

Design	N	Safety	Complexity	Power	Sel Prob	Utility

Table 12.4: Response-Adaptive Randomization Evaluation Matrix

Design	N	No. of Failures	Safety	Complexity	Power	Utility

Table 12.5: Dose-Escalation Design Evaluation Matrix

weight						
Design	Mean N	Mean DLTs	Mean MTD	SdMTD	Sel Prob	Utility

12.3.5   *Dose-Escalation Design*

Design input parameters: dose levels to explore, toxicity (response) model and prior distributions of the model parameters, DLT rate defined by the MTD, and stopping rules

Design outcome parameters (operating characteristics): mean number of patients required, mean DLTs, mean predicted MTD and standard deviation, selecting probabilities (this probability can be combined into the single index, Sel Prob, by using certain weights) (Table 12.5):

12.3.6   *Biomarker-Enrichment Design*

Design input parameters: the sample sizes for each stage for the biomarker positive and biomarker-negative populations; the maximum sample size; N, the treatment effects in biomarker positive and negative populations; and the standard deviation

Design outcome parameters (operating characteristics): the average sample size $\bar{N}$, the power for the biomarker positive population pPower, the power for the overpopulation, oPower, and the probability of rejecting the null hypothesis for either overpopulation or biomarker positive population (Table 12.6). The utility can be defined as

$$U = (N_+) pPower + (N_+ + N_-) oPower,$$

where N_+ and N_- are the size of biomarker positive and negative populations, respectively.

With the availability of a screening tool, the study complexity should also be considered.

Table 12.6: Biomarker-Enrichment Design Evaluation Matrix

Design	N̄	Power	pPower	oPower	Utility

Table 12.7: Biomarker-Informed Design Evaluation Matrix

Design	N	Power	Selection probabilities

12.3.7 *Biomarker-Informed Design*

Design input parameters: the parameters in the hierarchical biomarker model and sample size for each stage

Design outcome parameters (operating characteristics): power and selection probability for each arm (Table 12.7):

The optimal design to choose is the design with maximum utility.

Chapter 13

Monitoring Trials and Making Adaptations

After an adaptive trial starts, we need to monitor the trial and prepare for making adaptations based on interim analysis. Different adaptive designs have different adaptation rules, which we have discussed in previous chapters. Here we summarize them and provide necessary program tools.

13.1   Stopping and Arm-Selection

Group Sequential and Sample Size Reestimation Designs

For a group sequential, sample-size reestimation, drop-arm, and add-arm designs, the stopping boundaries are determined at the design stage. The trial monitoring procedure is to follow the predetermined stopping boundary at the design stage. Similarly, for CRM, we just need to follow the predetermined stopping rules (e.g., when the criterion of 6 patients at a dose level is reached).

Error-Spending Design

For a group sequential design with error-spending approach, when there is a change in the timing and/or the number of interim analyses, the stopping boundaries must be recalculated based on the predetermined error-spending function. The procedure is as if one designs a new trial with the new information time and/or the new number of analyses.

Pick-Winner Design

At the interim analysis, select the arm with the best response (or largest test statistic) and control arm to the second stage.

Adding-Arm Design

Stage 1: Pick the arm with the larger response (utility).

Stage 2: Add more arms and randomize the patients in terms of the threshold cR and cumulative responses in the new and initial arms.

13.2 Conditional Power

At the interim analysis, we often want to know the conditional power, which can be accomplished by invoking the R function in Appendix B. The following are examples of invoking the conditional power function:

ConPower(EP="binary", Model="MSP", alpha2=0.2050, ux=0.2, uy=0.4, nStg2=100, p1=0.1)

ConPower(EP="binary", Model="MPP", alpha2=0.0043, ux=0.2, uy=0.4, nStg2=100, p1=0.1)

ConPower(EP="binary", Model="MINP", alpha2=0.0226, ux=0.2, uy=0.4, nStg2=100, p1=0.1, w1=0.707)

ConPower(EP="normal", Model="MSP", alpha2=0.2050, ux=0.2, uy=0.4, sigma=1, nStg2=200, p1=0.1)

ConPower(EP="normal", Model="MPP", alpha2=0.0043, ux=0.2, uy=0.4, sigma=1, nStg2=200, p1=0.1)

ConPower(EP="normal", Model="MINP", alpha2=0.0226, ux=0.2, uy=0.4, sigma=1, nStg2=200, p1=0.1, w1=0.707)

13.3 Sample-Size Reestimation

For a sample-size reestimation design with MINP, the new sample size can be calculated using one of the following three methods:

New sample size for stage 2 by the maximum information design:

Given the interim sample size N_1, the new sample size required for the stage 2 is $N_2 = N - N_1$ or

$$N_2 = 2 \left(\frac{(\hat{\sigma}^*)^2}{\delta_0} - \frac{1}{4} \right) (z_{1-\alpha} + z_{1-\beta})^2 - N_1, \qquad (13.1)$$

where $(\hat{\sigma}^*)^2$ is "lumped variance" estimated at the interim analysis from the blinded data and δ_0 is the initial assessment for δ.

New sample size for stage 2 by the unblinded method:

$$n_2 = 2 \left(\frac{\hat{\sigma}}{\delta_0} \right)^2 \left[\frac{z_{1-\alpha} - w_1 z_{1-p_1}}{\sqrt{1-w_1^2}} - z_{1-cP} \right]^2, \qquad (13.2)$$

where δ_0 is the initial estimation of treatment difference and $(\hat{\sigma})^2$ is the variance estimated from the unblinded data at the interim analysis. Here the weight w_1 must be the same as that at the design stage.

New sample size for stage 2 by the mixed method:

$$n_2 = 2 \left(\frac{\hat{\sigma}^*}{\delta_0} \right)^2 \left[\frac{z_{1-\alpha} - w_1 z_{1-p_1}}{\sqrt{1 - w_1^2}} - z_{1-cP} \right]^2, \qquad (13.3)$$

where δ_0 is the initial estimation of treatment difference, $(\hat{\sigma}^*)^2$ is the variance estimated from the blinded data at the interim analysis, and the weight w_1 must be the same as at the design stage.

For two-stage unblinded SSR design with MSP, MPP, or MINP, the new sample size for the second stage can be obtained by invoking the R function "*NewN2byConditionalPowerForTwoStageSSR.*" Here is an example:

NewN2byConditionalPowerForTwoStageSSR(trtDiff=0.2, sigma=1.2, NId=0, p1=0.1, alpha2=0.0226, nStg2=50, cPower=0.9, method="MINP", w1=0.707)

13.4   New Randomization Scheme

Adaptive randomization changes as the observations are accumulating. It seems that we have to randomize the next patient as soon as the patient data are available, which is really inconvenient since a statistician who does the randomization has to wait 24/7. However, there is a simple solution: pregenerate 4 more randomized treatment codes for the next 2 patients with all possible outcome combinations. More conveniently we can use IVRS to generate if all the clinic sites can provide the patient data promptly.

Suppose we have observed responses of 11 patients, that is, ObsResponses=c(0,0,0,0,0,1,0,0,1,0,0), and we want to determine the dose level for the next patient. Here is the code with the CRM logistic model and the skeleton model. The results are: for the logistic model, the next patient (patient 12) should be assigned to dose level 2, while with the skeleton model the next patient should be assigned to dose level 6.

```
#Logistic Model
g= c(1); doses = c(1)
RRo = c(0.01,0.02,0.03,0.05,0.12,0.17,0.22,0.4)
ObsResponses=c(0,0,0,0,0,1,0,0,1,0,0)
for (k in 1:100) {g[k]=1}; # Flat prior
for (i in 1:8) {doses[i]=i}
CRM(nSims=500, nPts=11, nLevels=8, b=150, aMin=0, aMax=3,
MTRate=0.17, ToxModel="Logist", nPtsForStop=6)
#Skeleton Model
g = c(1); doses = c(1)
```

RRo = c(0.01,0.02,0.03,0.05,0.12,0.17,0.22,0.4)
skeletonP=c(0.01,0.02,0.04,0.08,0.16,0.32,0.4,0.5)
ObsResponses=c(0,0,0,0,0,1,0,0,1,0,0)
for (k in 1:100) {g[k]=1}; # Flat prior
CRM(nSims=500, nPts=11, nLevels=8, aMin=-0.1, aMax=2,
MTRate=0.17, ToxModel="Skeleton", nPtsForStop=6)

We can prepare the randomization code for the 13th and 14th patients by running the CRM monitoring code with two possible responses for the 12th and 13th patients. For example, to generate two possible dose levels for the 13th patient, we need to use ObsResponses=c(0,0,0,0,0,1,0,0,1,0,0,0), ObsResponses=c(0,0,0,0,0,1,0,0,1,0,0,1) to run the simulation twice. If we use an IVRS, we can randomize the patient at real time.

Response-Adaptive Randomization

For a two-arm design with a binary endpoint, the randomization probability is

$$\Pr(trt = i) = \frac{n_i}{n_1 + n_2}. \tag{13.4}$$

In general, the allocation probability is given by

$$\Pr(trt = i) = \frac{H(\hat{u}_i - \hat{u}_{\max} + \delta_{NI})}{\sum_{i=1}^{M} H(\hat{u}_i - \hat{u}_{\max} + \delta_{NI})}. \tag{13.5}$$

Chapter 14

Data Analyses of Adaptive Trials

14.1 Orderings in Sample Space

Data analyses of an adaptive trial include point and confidence parameter estimates, and adjusted (conditional and unconditional) p-values. The issues surrounding these topics are controversial; even the definition of bias, confidence interval, and p-value are not unique with adaptive trials.

Unlike the bias in a classical trial without adaptation, the concept of bias in adaptive trials is complicated. For example, the first kind of bias concerns the unconditional estimate: Suppose a particular adaptive trial is repeated for infinite times; the unconditional treatment effect is defined as the expected mean treatment differences between the two treatment groups over all the trials regardless of whether the trial is stopped at an interim stage or at the final stage. The difference between the expected mean difference and the truth treatment difference is the bias. We may say that this view of bias is from statisticians' perspective because the statistician can possibly see all these results. The second bias concerns the estimate (called stagewise conditional estimate) conditional on the stage where the trial stopped. Imagine that the trial is repeated infinitely; we estimate the treatment effect by averaging the mean treatment differences over all the trials that stopped at any given stage. The third kind of bias concerns the estimate conditional on the positive results (e.g., mean differences that are statistically significant). Such an estimate of treatment effect can be considered as the regulatory view or patients' view because they usually see only such positive results. The bias of such conditional estimates also directly relates the publication bias. This type of bias also exists in classical design with a fixed sample size.

The stagewise conditional estimate is most often studied in the statistical community and is also the focus of this chapter. It is interesting to know that we aggregate all type-I errors from different stages and controlled at an α level, but the conditional estimate only concerns the possible results at the stage where the trial actually stopped.

When the null hypothesis H_0 is true, $f^a(t) = f^o(t)$, p-value P has a uniform distribution in $[0, 1]$. However, p-value from an adaptive trial does not have this nice property. Not only that, the p-value, median, and confidence limits depend on ordering the sample space (k, z), where k is the stage number and z is the standardized Z statistic. For instance, at the end of a classical clinical trial, a test statistic $z_1 = 2.3$ is more extreme than $z_2 = 1.8$. In other words, the value of test statistics alone is sufficient to determine the "extremeness" or the sample space orderings. However, in adaptive trials, the definition of extremeness or the ordering is much more complicated; it requires at least a pair of values (k, z). Suppose, in a two-stage group sequential trial with $H_0 : \mu \leq 0$ versus $H_a : \mu > 0$, that O'Brien-Fleming stopping boundaries with equal information time $(z_{1-\alpha_1} = 2.8$ and $z_{1-\alpha_2} = 1.98)$ are used. If we observed the test statistic $z_1 = 2.5$ at the first stage and $z_2 = 2.0$ at the second stage, which value is more extreme? At the first look, we may think z_1 is more extreme because z_1 is larger than z_2, but according to the stopping boundaries, we don't reject H_0 at the first stage but reject it at the second stage. Therefore, it is reasonable to consider the pair data $(k, z) = (2, 2.0)$ more extreme than the pair data $(1, 2.5)$. On the other hand, if the Pocock boundaries $(z_{1-\alpha_1} = 2.18$ and $z_{1-\alpha_2} = 2.18)$ are used, we can say z_1 is more extreme than z_2 because we reject H_0 at the first stage. After we define the orderings in the sample space, we can define the p-value. That is, with the observed pair of statistics (k_0, z_0) when the trial is stopped, a one-sided upper p-value can be computed as

$$\Pr_{\theta=0} \{(k, z) \succeq (k_0, z_0)\}. \tag{14.1}$$

It is obvious that definition of sample space ordering (denoted by $\succeq$) is somewhat subjective. It can be one of the following:

Stagewise Ordering

If the continuation regions of a design are intervals, the stagewise ordering (Fairbanks and Madsen, 1982; Tsiatis, Rosner, and Mehta, 1984; Jennison and Turnbull, 2000, pp. 179–180) uses counterclockwise ordering around the continuation region to compute the p-value, unbiased median estimate, and confidence limits. This ordering depends on the stopping region, stopping stage, information time at interim analyses, and standardized statistic at the stopping stage. But it does not depend on information levels beyond the observed stage. For a one-sided design with an upper alternative, $(k', z') \succeq (k_0, z_0)$, if one of the following criteria holds: (1) $k = k'$ and $z' > z$, (2) $k' < k$ and $z' \geq a_{k'}$, the upper efficacy boundary at stage k' and (3) $k' > k$ and $z' < b_k$, the upper futility boundary at stage k.

Likelihood Ratio Ordering

The likelihood ratio (LR) ordering (Chang, 1989) depends on the observed standardized Z statistic z, information levels, and a specified hypothetical reference. For the LR ordering under a given hypothesis $H_a : \theta = \theta_g$, we have $(k', z') \succ (k, z)$ if $\left(z' - \theta_g \sqrt{\tau_{k'}} \right) > \left(z - \theta_g \sqrt{\tau_k} \right)$. Under the null hypothesis $H_0 : \theta = 0$, it reduces to $z' > z$ and can be used to derive statistics under H_0, such as p-values.

The LR ordering is applicable to all designs if all information levels are available. But depending on the boundary shape, some observed statistics (k, z) in the rejection region might be less extreme than the statistics in the acceptance region. That is, the p-value for observed statistics in the rejection region might be greater than the significance level.

Maximum Likelihood Estimate Ordering

The maximum likelihood estimate (MLE) ordering (Emerson and Fleming, 1990) depends only on the observed maximum likelihood estimate. We have $(k', z') \succ (k, z)$ if $\frac{z'}{\sqrt{k'}} > \frac{z}{\sqrt{k}}$. The MLE ordering is applicable to all designs if all information levels are available.

Score Test Ordering

The score test ordering (Rosner and Tsiatis, 1988) is to rank the outcomes by values of the score statistic for testing $H_0 : \theta = 0$. That is, $(k', z') \succ (k, z)$ if $z' \sqrt{k'} > z \sqrt{k}$.

14.2 Adjusted p-Value

14.2.1 *Definitions of p-Values*

The p-value for test H_0 on observing (k^*, z^*) is defined as

$$\Pr \left\{ \text{Obtain } (k, z) \succeq (k^*, z^*) | H_0 \right\}, \qquad (14.2)$$

where $\succeq$ means "as extreme as or more extreme than," where the ordering is defined in the previous section.

Alternatively, we can define the conditional p-value as

$$\Pr \left\{ \text{Obtain } z \geq z^* \right) | H_0, k \right\}. \qquad (14.3)$$

14.2.2 *Simulation Approach*

Running the trial N times under H_0, obtain the number of times (n) of the calculated test statistic $\succeq$ the observed value based on the orderings in sample space. The p-value is $p = n/N$.

Suppose the test value z^* is observed at stage k, the conditional p-value can be obtained by running the trial N times under H_0, among which M times the trials stopped at stage k, and among the M times, there are n times that the calculated test statistics are larger than or equal to z^*. The conditional p-value at stage k is $p_c = n/M$. As an example, we provide R function: p-value by simulation, in Appendix B and an application below.

Taking Example 3.1 for instance, suppose we observed test statistic $t_2 = 1.96$ at stage 2; the simulation gives the stagewise-ordering p-value of 0.0305 and conditional p-value = 0.0205.

Here is the code to invoke the R function for the p-value simulation:

```
## Example 14.1
PvalueTwoStageGSDwithNormalEndpoint(u0=0.05,u1=0.05,
sigma0=0.22, sigma1=0.22, n0Stg1=120, n1Stg1=120, n0Stg2=120, n1Stg2=120,
alpha1=0.01, t2Obs=1.96)
```

14.3   Parameter Estimation

Consider the hypothesis test for mean μ:

$$H_0 : \mu \leq 0 \text{ versus } H_a : \mu > 0.$$

Let x_{ik} be the independent observations from the ith patient at the kth stage ($k = 1, 2$). Assume x_{ik} has the normal distribution $N\left(\mu, \sigma^2\right)$ with known σ. Denote by $\bar{x}_k$ the stagewise sample mean at the kth stage (not based on cumulative data); thus $\bar{x}_1$ and $\bar{x}_2$ are independent in a GSD. The test statistic at the first stage of the standard group sequential design can be written as $T_1 = \bar{x}_1\sqrt{n_1}/\sigma$, where n_1 is the sample size at the first stage. For a group sequential design with futility stopping boundary c_0, and efficacy stopping boundary c_1 on the z-scale, the bias is (Emerson, 1988; Jennison and Turnbull, 2000, p. 177)

$$\Delta_{bias} = \mu_{MLE} - \mu = \frac{n_2\sigma}{(n_1 + n_2)\sqrt{n_1}} \left\{ \phi\left(c_0 - \frac{\mu}{\sigma}\sqrt{n_1}\right) - \phi\left(c_1 - \frac{\mu}{\sigma}\sqrt{n_1}\right)\right\},$$
(14.4)

where ϕ is the standard normal p.d.f.

To calculate μ_1 and μ_2, the standard normal c.d.f. can be approximated by

$$\Phi_0(c) = 1 - \frac{(c^2 + 5.575192695c + 12.77436324)\exp\left(-c^2/2\right)}{\sqrt{2\pi}c^3 + 14.38718147c^2 + 31.53531977c + 2(12.77436324)}.$$
(14.5)

Since the bias is a function true parameter μ we can use an iterative method to obtain the unbiased estimate of μ. That is, $\hat{\mu} = \mu + Bias\,(\mu)$; we use $\hat{\mu}^{(k)} = \mu + Bias\left(\hat{\mu}^{(k-1)}\right)$, where $\hat{\mu}^{(k)}$ is the kth iterative value and $\mu^{(0)} = \bar{X}$.

For a given GSD, one can run N sets of simulations. In each set of simulations (with M runs) a different treatment difference is used and the average or MLE of treatment difference is obtained. Thus for each set of simulations we have a pair of data consisting of true difference and average difference; we then plot a curve through N pair of these data. With this plot we can obtain a unbiased estimate simply by finding the true mean based on the MLE mean in the clinical trial.

14.4   Confidence Interval

The confidence interval calculation is usually complicated for adaptive designs. There are even several different definitions of confidence intervals dependent on the sample space orderings.

Recall that for the classical design without any adaptations and the hypothesis $H_0 : \mu \leq \mu_0$, the $100(1-\alpha)\%$ one-sided confidence interval of μ can be defined as all the values of μ_0 such that H_0 will not be rejected, given observed data z. For a group sequential design, we can take the similar approach; we can find a pair $(k_u(\mu_0), z_u(\mu_0))$ such that

$$\Pr_{\mu=\mu_0} \{(T, Z_T) \succeq (k_u(\mu_0), z_u(\mu_0))\} = \alpha. \tag{14.6}$$

Then, the acceptance region

$$A(\mu_0) = \{(k, z) : (k, z) \prec (k_u(\mu_0), z_u(\mu_0))\} \tag{14.7}$$

defines a one-sided hypothesis test of $H_0 : \mu \leq \mu_0$ with type-I error rate α. The $100(1-\alpha)\%$ one-sided confidence set contains all values μ_0 for which the hypothesis $H_0 : \mu \leq \mu_0$ is accepted. The confidence set is not necessarily a continuous region.

The so-called repeated confidence interval at the k, RCI_k, consists of all possible values for the parameter for which the null hypothesis will not be rejected given the observed value. When x_{ij} is normally distributed and MINP is used in a GSD, the RCI_k can be expressed as

$$(\bar{x} - c_k \sigma_{\bar{x}}, \bar{x} + c_k \sigma_{\bar{x}}), \tag{14.8}$$

in which c_k is the stopping boundary at the kth stage and $\sigma_{\bar{x}}$ is the standard deviation of $\bar{x}$.

A general approach to obtain RCI_k numerically is through Monte Carlo simulations, but we are not going to discuss the simulation details here.

14.5   Summary

We have discussed the analyses following an adaptive trial, including the p-value, parameter estimation, and confidence interval. We see that there are controversies surrounding such analyses, mainly because these quantities are dependent on the sample space (conditional or unconditional sample space) and sample space orderings. As a result, there are different versions of p-values and confidence intervals, which make the clinical interpretations very difficult. The estimation bias and variance of the estimation are definitely a trade-off in adaptive design settings. We should balance these two aspects and clinical interpretations as well. In the current practice, the naive, sample mean or MLE is still a common estimation; unadjusted p-values and unadjusted confidence intervals are still common outcomes reported for an adaptive trial.

Chapter 15

Planning and Execution

The US FDA released the draft Guidance for Industry, Adaptive Design Clinical Trials for Drugs and Biologics in February 2010. Since then, more than four years have passed, and no updated or final version has been seen yet. Because it is a draft, it is not recommended for implementation. Adaptive design study has made big progress in the past five years and some of the FDA's views in the draft may be out of date. Nevertheless, there is much valuable information of which we should be aware and everyone who practices adaptive trials should carefully read the draft guidance. The *Journal of Biopharmaceutical Statistics* published a special issue (Liu and Chang, 2010) of discussion papers on the draft adaptive design guidance. In this special discussion issue, technical papers are invited not only to address existing problems with adaptive designs as pointed out by the FDA guidance but also to introduce new designs for clinical trial settings that have not been adequately tackled in the literature.

15.1 Study Planning

Before the implementation of an adaptive design, it is recommended that the following practical issues be considered. First, determine whether an adaptive design is feasible for the intended trial. For example, will the adaptive design require extraordinary efforts for implementation? Are the level of difficulty and the associated cost justifiable for the gain from the adaptive design? Will the implementation of the adaptive design delay patient recruitment and prolong the duration of the study? Would delayed responses diminish the advantage of the adaptive design? How often will the unblinded analyses be practical, and to whom should the data be unblinded? How should the impact of a Data Monitoring Committee's (DMC's) decisions regarding the trial (e.g., recommending early stopping or other adaptations due to safety concerns) be considered at the design stage? Second, we should ensure the validity of the adaptive design for the intended trial. For example, will the unblinding cause potential bias in treatment assessment? Will the implementation of the adaptive design destroy the randomness? Third, we should have an expectation about the degree of flexibility (sensitivity or robustness). For example, will protocol deviations or violations invalidate the adaptive method? How might an unexpected DMC action affect the power and validity of the design? In designing a trial, we should also consider how to prevent premature release of the interim results to the general public using information masks because releasing information could affect the rest of the trial and endanger the integrity of the trial. Regarding study design, we strongly suggest early communication with the regulatory agency and DMC regarding the study protocol and the DMC charter. For broader discussions of planning different adaptive designs, please see the PhRMA full white papers on adaptive design (Quinlan, Gallo, and Krams, 2006; Gallo, 2006, Gaydos et al., 2006; Maca et al., 2006; Chuang et al., 2006)

Traditional drug development is subjective to a large extent, and intuitive decision-making processes are primarily based on individual experiences. Therefore, optimal design is often not achieved. Clinical trial simulation (CTS) is a powerful tool for providing an objective evaluation of development plans and study designs for program optimization and for supporting strategic decision-making. CTS is very intuitive and easy to implement with minimal cost and can be done in a short time. The utilities of CTS include but are not limited to (1) sensitivity analysis and risk assessment; (2) estimation of probability of success (power); (3) design evaluation and optimization; (4) cost, time, and risk reduction; (5) clinical development program evaluation and prioritization; (6) trial monitoring and interim prediction of future outcomes; (7) prediction of long-term benefit using short-term outcomes; (8) validation of trial design and statistical methods; and (9) streamlining communication among different parties. Within regulatory bodies, CTS has been frequently used for assessing the robustness of results, validating statistical methodology, and predicting long-term benefit in accelerated approvals. CTS plays an important role in adaptive design for the following reasons: First, statistical theory for adaptive designs is often complicated under some relatively strong assumptions, and CTS is useful in modeling very complicated situations with minimum assumptions not only to control type-I error, but also to calculate the power, and to generate many other important operating characteristics such as the expected sample-size, conditional power, and unbiased estimates. Second, CTS can be used to evaluate the robustness of the adaptive design against protocol deviations. Moreover, CTS can be used as a tool to monitor trials, predict outcomes, identify potential problems, and provide remedies for resolutions during the conduct of the trials.

In summary, clinical trial simulation is a useful tool for adaptive designs in clinical research. It can help investigators achieve better planning, better designs, better monitoring, and generally better execution of clinical trials. In addition, it can help to (1) streamline the drug development process, (2) increase the probability of success, and (3) reduce the cost and time-to-market in pharmaceutical research and development.

15.2 Working with a Regulatory Agency

It is important to assure the validity of the adaptive design. Companies should begin a dialogue about adaptive designs with FDA medical officers and statisticians as early as a year before beginning a trial. Dr. O'Neill from the FDA said (The Pink Sheet, Dec. 18, 2006, p. 24), "We're most concerned about estimating what you think you are estimating." Is the hypothesis testing appropriate? Do you know what you are rejecting at end of day? Can you say you are controlling the false positive?"

Another reason to communicate with the agency early is that the FDA could be of assistance in sharing the data or at least the disease information or models. Building off external data and experience is sometimes a crucial element of adaptive design.

The FDA released the draft guidance for Adaptive Design Clinical Trials for Drugs and Biologics in 2010. This guidance gives advice on topics such as (1) what aspects of adaptive design trials (i.e., clinical, statistical, regulatory) call for special consideration, (2) when to interact with FDA while planning and conducting adaptive design studies, (3) what information to include in the adaptive design for FDA review, and (4) issues to consider in the evaluation of a completed adaptive design study. This guidance is intended to assist sponsors in planning and conducting adaptive design clinical studies, and to facilitate an efficient FDA review (FDA, 2010).

FDA's guidance describes the Agency's current thinking on a topic and should be viewed only as recommendations, not requirements. In the guidance, an adaptive design clinical study is defined as a study that includes a prospectively planned opportunity for modification of one or more specified aspects of the study design and hypotheses based on analysis of data (usually interim data) from subjects in the study. Analyses of the accumulating study data are performed at prospectively planned timepoints within the study, can be performed in a fully blinded manner or in an unblinded manner, and can occur with or without formal statistical hypothesis testing.

The adaptations include but are not limited to:

- Study eligibility criteria (either for subsequent study enrollment or for a subset selection of an analytic population)
- Randomization procedure

- Treatment regimens of the different study groups (e.g., dose level, schedule, duration)
- Total sample size of the study (including early termination)
- Concomitant treatments used
- Planned schedule of patient evaluations for data collection (e.g., number of intermediate timepoints, timing of last patient observation, and duration of patient study participation)
- Primary endpoint (e.g., which of several types of outcome assessments, which timepoint of assessment, use of a unitary versus composite endpoint, or the components included in a composite endpoint)
- Election and/or order of secondary endpoints
- Analytic methods to evaluate the endpoints (e.g., covariates of final analysis, statistical methodology, type-I error control)

The FDA raises two main concerns with adaptive design: (1) whether the adaptation process has led to design, analysis, or conduct flaws that have introduced bias that increases the chance of a false conclusion that the treatment is effective (a type-I error) and (2) whether the adaptation process has led to positive study results that are difficult to interpret irrespective of having control of type-I error.

The FDA classifies general adaptive designs into two categories: well-understood and less well-understood adaptive designs. The well-understood adaptive designs include:

(1) Adaptation of study eligibility criteria based on analyses of pretreatment (baseline) data
(2) Adaptations to maintain study power based on blinded interim analyses of aggregate data
(3) Adaptations based on interim results of an outcome unrelated to efficacy
(4) Adaptations using group sequential methods and the drop-loser designs
(5) Adaptations in the data analysis plan not dependent on within-study, between-group outcome differences

As suggested in the guidance, a blinded SSR design with a binary, survival, or continuous endpoint requires no alpha adjustment. However, as we have discussed, the unblinded SSR can inflate the alpha to some degree.

For drop-loser designs, the FDA states that studies with multiple groups (e.g., multiple-dose levels) can be designed to carry only one or two groups to completion out of the several initiated, based on this type of futility analysis done by group. One or more unblinded interim analyses of the apparent treatment effect in each group is examined, and groups that meet the prospective futility criterion are terminated. However, because of the multiplicity arising from the several sequential interim analyses over time with multiple between-group analyses done to select groups to discontinue, statistical adjustments and the usual group sequential alpha spending adjustments need to be made in this case to control type-I error rates.

The guidance stated: "For the group sequential methods to be valid, it is important to adhere to the prospective analytic plan, terminating the group if a futility criterion is met, and not terminating the study for efficacy unless the prospective efficacy criterion is achieved. Failure to follow the prospective plan in either manner risks confounding interpretation of the study results." This seems to suggest a futility bonding rule. If it indeed is, a bigger alpha can be used for the group design with a futility boundary.

The less well understood adaptive designs include:

(1) Adaptations for dose selection studies
(2) Adaptive randomization based on relative treatment group responses
(3) Adaptation of sample size based on interim-effect size estimates
(4) Adaptation of patient population based on treatment-effect estimates
(5) Adaptation for endpoint selection based on interim estimate of treatment effect
(6) Adaptations in noninferiority studies

Generally, adaptive designs with well-understood properties can get the FDA blessing earlier than less well-understood designs. However, the draft guidance released four years ago. During those four years, research and practice of adaptive designs have made progress. Some designs understood yesterday may become well-understood today.

Regarding the interaction with the FDA when planning and conducting an adaptive design, the FDA stated that the purpose and nature of the interactions between a study sponsor and FDA varies with the study's location (stage) within the drug development program. The increased complexity of some adaptive design studies and uncertainties regarding their performance characteristics may warrant earlier and more extensive interactions than usual. In general, the FDA encourages adaptive designs in early and middle periods of drug development, but suggests cational use in late stages of drug development.

The FDA will generally not be involved in examining the interim data used for the adaptive decision-making and will not provide comments on the adaptive decisions while the study is ongoing. FDA's review and acceptance at the protocol design stage of the methodology for the adaptation process does not imply its advance concurrence that the adaptively selected choices will be the optimal choices. Special protocol assessments (SPAs) entail timelines (45-day responses) and commitments that may not be best suited for adaptive design studies. The full review and assessment of a study using less well-understood adaptive design methods can be complex, will involve a multidisciplinary evaluation team, and might involve extended discussions among individuals within different FDA offices before reaching a conclusion. If there has been little or no prior discussion between FDA and the study sponsor regarding the proposed study and its adaptive design features, other information requests following initial FDA evaluation are likely and full completion of study assessment within the SPA 45-day time frame is unlikely. Sponsors are therefore encouraged to have thorough discussions with the FDA regarding the study design and the study's place within the development program before considering submitting an SPA request.

15.3   Trial Execution

15.3.1   *Dynamic Drug Supply*

Conventional Drug Supply

The conventional way for drug supply in a clinical trial separates the supply chains for each stratum or treatment group. In this approach, an initial drug shipment would be made for each stratum. Resupply shipments would then follow, based on fixed trigger levels for each stratum. However, keeping the supply chains separate requires a high initial outlay and can result in a lot of waste if a site does not enroll as anticipated. This conventional drug supply can be particularly problematic for adaptive trials.

As Hamilton and Ho (2004) described, to randomize a patient, a site would call the IVRS and enter some basic patient identifiers such as ID number and date of birth, along with the stratum to which the patient belonged. The system would then access the randomization and treatment kit lists and read back to site personnel the blinded kit number assigned to that patient. A fax confirming patient information and assigned kit number would then be automatically generated by the system and sent to the site.

Dynamic Drug Supply

Stratified and adaptive randomizations place a challenge on drug supply because the randomization list can't be predetermined. A conventional supply algorithm based on site is often overly conservative and a potentially waste drug.

To reduce waste in the drug supply process, efforts have been devoted to the use of interactive voice response systems (IVRSs) combined with allocation algorithms, as well as package design options. McEntegart (2003) proposed a scheme to force subject randomization into treatments for which stocks of medication are available. Dowlman (2001) describes savings that can be achieved if medications are not linked to subject numbers until the point of dispensation. Hamilton and Ho (2004) proposed a dynamic drug supply algorithm based on a patient-coverage concept and demonstrated through simulation a significant saving on drug supply.

Case Study 15.1: Dynamic Drug Supply

Hamilton and Ho (2004) deal with a clinical study requiring stratification. In the initial planning stages for this study, it was determined that there would not be enough drug supply for clinic sites according to the conventional seeding. They develop a more efficient algorithm for drug supply in terms of patient coverage, as opposed to the amount of medication remaining at each site. They focused on two key questions: (1) how much drug is required in order to randomize the next y patients, regardless of strata; and (2) given the current level of drug on hand, how many more patients can be randomized.

Their logistic steps for the dynamic supply are:

(1) At site initiation, ship enough drug to cover the first y patients enrolling into the study, regardless of strata.
(2) After each patient is randomized, recalculate the patient coverage based on the randomization list and current levels of drug supply at the site.
(3) If the patient coverage falls below a lower resupply threshold x, ship enough drug to replenish supplies to an upper resupply threshold y. That is, ship enough drug so that the next y patients can be enrolled into the study, regardless of strata.

The implementation aspect of the dynamic supply can be further elaborated as follows: In the original study, the dynamic drug supply scheme was implemented utilizing a telephone-based interactive voice response system (Figure 15.1). The system was designed in such a way that when a site completed regulatory and contractual requirements, sponsor personnel could go to a secure administrative web page and activate that site. Upon activation, the system would examine the randomization list for that site and calculate the amount of drug needed to cover the first y patients, regardless of strata. Notifications via email and fax would then be sent to the central drug repository indicating which drug kits to ship and the shipment number to appear on the waybill. When the site received the drug shipment, they were instructed to register the shipment number with the IVRS, making those drug kits available to be used to randomize patients at the site.

The steps to randomize a patient via IVRS are similar to the conversional approach. After each patient was successfully randomized, the IVRS would recalculate patient coverage at the site. If patient coverage dropped below x patients, another calculation was made by the IVRS to determine which kit types were necessary to bring the coverage back up to cover the next y patients. An automatic notification would then be sent to the central drug repository, indicating the drug kits to be shipped to the site.

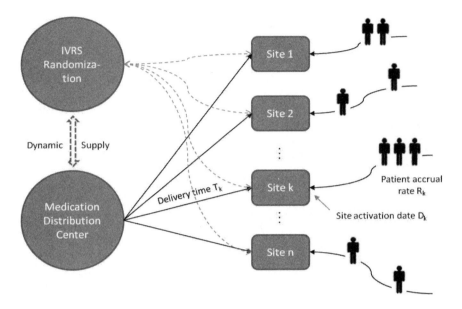

Figure 15.1:   Sketch of Dynamic Medication Supply System

15.3.2   *Data Monitor Committee*

Necessities of Trial Monitoring

To protect the integrity of a clinical trial, data monitoring is necessary. The monitoring, often carried out by an independent data monitor committee (DMC), includes safety and/or efficacy aspects.

As pointed in FDA guidance (FDA, 2006), all clinical trials require safety monitoring, but not all trials require monitoring by a formal committee that may be external to the trial organizers, sponsors, and investigators. Data monitor committees (DMCs) have generally been established for large, randomized multisite studies that evaluate treatments intended to prolong life or reduce risk of a major adverse health outcome such as a cardiovascular event or recurrence of cancer. DMCs are generally recommended for any controlled trial of any size that will compare rates of mortality or major morbidity, but a DMC is not required or recommended for most clinical studies. DMCs are generally not needed, for example, for trials at early stages of product development. They are also generally not needed for trials addressing lesser outcomes, such as relief of symptoms, unless the trial population is at elevated risk of more severe outcomes.

To have a DMC will add administrative complexity to a trial and require additional resources, so we recommend that sponsors limit the use of a DMC to the circumstances. The FDA guidance describes, mainly from a safety perspective, several factors to consider when determining whether to establish a

DMC (more commonly used name is DSMB – Data Safety Monitoring Board) for a particular trial. Particularly, the FDA suggests using a DMC when:

(1) The study endpoint is such that a highly favorable or unfavorable result, or even a finding of futility, at an interim analysis might ethically require termination of the study before its planned completion;
(2) There are prior reasons for a particular safety concern, as, for example, if the procedure for administering the treatment is particularly invasive;
(3) There is prior information suggesting the possibility of serious toxicity with the study treatment;
(4) The study is being performed in a potentially fragile population such as children, pregnant women or the very elderly, or other vulnerable populations, such as those who are terminally ill or of diminished mental capacity;
(5) The study is being performed in a population at elevated risk of death or other serious outcomes, even when the study objective addresses a lesser endpoint;
(6) The study is large, of long duration, and multicenter.

Keep in mind that clinical trial investigators or physicians monitor the patients on individual bases, whereas the DMC review focuses on the aggregated data and safety trends with respect to the treatment(s).

So far, there is no official guidance from the FDA regarding interim analysis monitoring for an adaptive design, which will take both efficacy and safety into consideration. In adaptive design, "benefit-risk ratio" is the key factor for interim decision making. When considering both efficacy and safety, there are common issues that affect a DMC's decision, such as short-term versus long-term treatment effects, early termination philosophies, response to early beneficial trends, response to early unfavorable trends, and response where there are no apparent trends (Ellenberg, Fleming, and DeMets, 2002; Pocock, 2005). It is recommended that a DMC be established to monitor the trial when an adaptive design is employed in clinical trials, especially when many adaptations are considered for allowing greater flexibility.

The stopping rule chosen in the design phase serves as a guideline to a DMC (Ellenberg, Fleming, and DeMets, 2002) as it makes a decision to recommend continuing or stopping a clinical trial. If all aspects of the conduct of the clinical trial adhered exactly to the conditions stipulated during the design phase, the stopping rule obtained during the design phase could be used directly. However, there are usually complicating factors that must be dealt with during the conduct of the trial.

DMC meetings are typically based on the availability of its members, which may be different from the schedules set at the design stage. The enrollment may be different from the assumption made at the design phase. Deviation in the analysis schedule may affect the stopping boundaries; therefore, the boundaries may need to be recalculated based on the actual schedules.

The true variability of the response variable is never known, but the actual data collected at interim analysis may show that the initial estimates in the design phase are inaccurate. Deviation in the variability estimation could affect the stopping boundaries. In this case, we may want to know the likelihood of success of the trial based on current data available, known as conditional power. Similarly, the treatment effect may be different from the initial estimation. This can lead to an adaptive design or sample-size reestimation (Chapter 5).

Data Monitor Committee Charter

The monitoring of a clinical trial for scientific integrity is a dual responsibility of the DMC and the sponsor. The DMC charter, developed and approved by the sponsor and DMC, is a central document for the monitoring. The DMC charter explicitly defines the roles and responsibilities of the DMC and describes the procedures to be used in carrying out its functions such as meeting frequency and format, and voting procedures as well. The DMC charter serves to delineate and make explicit the various responsibilities of the sponsor, the DMC, and other parties (e.g., CROs) involved.

There are different versions of DMC charters. However, the key contents are more or less the same. The following structure of a DMC charter is adapted from Fisher and colleagues (2001).

- Overview of IDMC Responsibilities:

    - Ethical responsibilities to study participants to monitor safety and efficacy
    - Scientific responsibilities to investigators and sponsors to monitor scientific integrity of the trial
    - Economic responsibilities to the sponsor to monitor the trial for futility

- Organization:

    - Composition
    - Selection of members

- Specific Functions:

    - Review the study protocol and any protocol amendments
    - Review data collection methods and safety monitoring procedures
    - Review and approve the DMC charter
    - Review and approve an interim analysis plan
    - Review interim monitoring reports and make recommendations to the steering committee

- Responsibilities of the Sponsor:

  - Make resources and information, including study documents, available to the DMC as necessary to carry out its designated functions
  - Monitor the study conduct and the collection and quality control of study data
  - Contract with the CRO for the preparation of interim monitoring reports
  - Inform the IDMC of any potential safety concern that is idiosyncratic or previously unreported
  - Provide analysis sets to the SAC containing data necessary for preparing DMC reports
  - Handle, financially and logistically, meeting arrangements of the DMC
  - Communicate regulatory information to relevant authorities

- Responsibilities of the CRO:

  - Prepare and distribute a draft DMC charter
  - Prepare and distribute a draft interim analysis plan
  - Prepare and distribute study reports based on data received from the sponsor
  - Prepare summary notes of each DMC meeting or conference call

- Conduct of DMC Meetings:

  - Meeting frequency and format (e.g., open, closed, executive sessions)
  - Definition of quorum and voting procedures
  - Procedures for recommendations to the steering committee
  - Summary notes
  - Confidentiality requirements
  - Conflict of interest guidelines

- Appendix I – Statistical Interim Monitoring Guidelines
- Appendix II – General Considerations for Early Termination

15.4 Summary

Adaptive design methods represent new territory in drug development. Using adaptive design, we can increase the chances for the success of a trial with reduced cost. Bayesian approaches provide new tools for optimizing trial design and clinical development program planning by integrating all the relevant knowledge and information available. Clinical trial simulations offer a powerful tool to design and monitor trials. The combination of adaptive design, the Bayesian approach, and trial simulation forms an ultimate statistical instrument for most successful drug development programs.

Appendix A

Thirty-Minute Tutorial to R

A.1 Introduction

R is a freeware system; you can download it onto your own PC. To install R, go to the website

http://cran.r-project.org/doc/manuals/r-release/R-admin.html

and choose hyperlink according to your operation system (Windows, Mac, or Unix). Follow the simple instructions to install R on your PC.

What is R? According to the official website, R is a language and environment for statistical computing and graphics. R provides a wide variety of statistical and graphical techniques, and is highly extensible. One of R's strengths is the ease with which well-designed publication-quality plots can be produced, including mathematical symbols and formulae where needed.

R is available as free software under the terms of the Free Software Foundation's GNU General Public License in source code form. It compiles and runs on a wide variety of UNIX platforms and similar systems (including FreeBSD and Linux), Windows, and MacOS.

You can type your commands or code directly at the command prompt ">" as shown in Figure A.1, or you may type somewhere else and when you finish it then copy and paste it in the command prompt. For instance, you can click manual *File->New* Script to create a line of R code and then save it for future use or open an existing R program file by clicking *File->Open* and choosing the desired file. The file saved from this R Editor will have the extension "R."

When you work in R you create objects that are stored in the current workspace. Each object created remains in the image unless you explicitly delete it. You can save the workspace at any time by clicking on the disc icon at the top of the control panel.

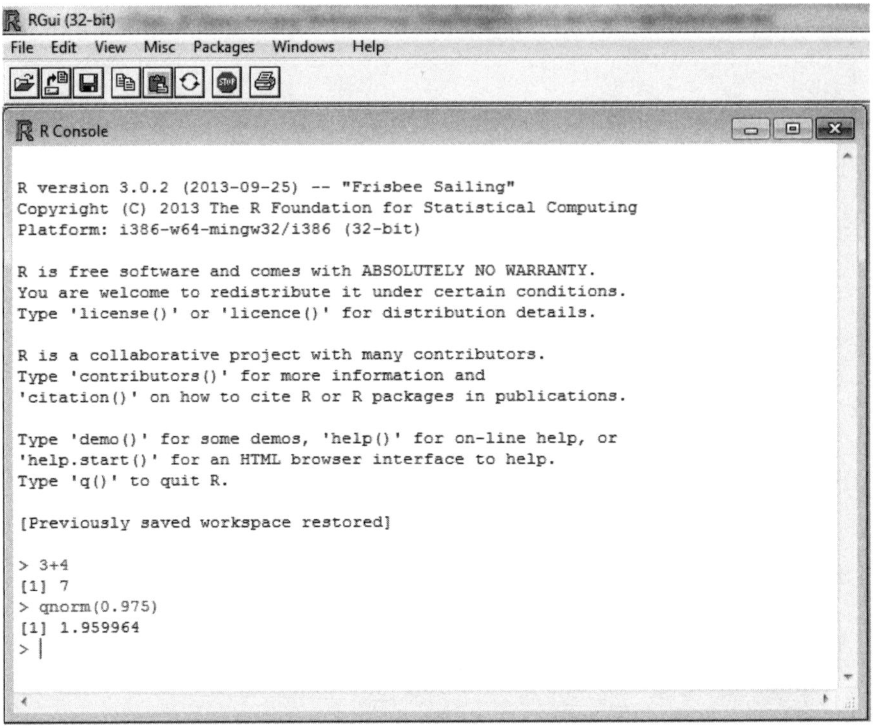

Figure A.1:   R Workspace with Examples of 3+4 and a Normal Percentile

A.2   R Language Basics

R stores information and operates on objects. The simplest objects are scalars, vectors, and matrices. But there are many others: lists and dataframes, for example. In advanced use of R it can also be useful to define new types of objects, specific for particular applications. We will stick with just the most commonly used objects here.

A.2.1   *Arithmetics*

If you type:
> 4+6*2
you will get the result:
[1] 16

Two or more statements can be written in a single line but separated by a semicolon. For example, if your inputs are
> x=-6; y=-4*3

> -x+y

the output will be

[1] -6

A.2.2 *Vector*

A example of vector is

> rep(0,4)

[1] 0 0 0 0

Another example is

> x=c(1,2,4); y=c(2,0,1); x+y

[1] 3 2 5

A.2.3 *Matrix*

Here is a simple example of matrix:

> x=c(1,3); y=c(2,1); cbind(x,y)

    x y

[1,] 1 2

[2,] 3 1

A.2.4 *Functions*

R has many built-in functions that are packed into groups, called packages. Commonly used functions are loaded automatically; to use other functions you may have to load the corresponding packages.

The examples of commonly used functions are:

> x=c(1,2,4,0,2.5,3.6,2,4)

> mean(x)

[1] 2.3875

> var(x)

[1] 2.086964

> summary(x)

 Min. 1st Qu. Median Mean 3rd Qu. Max.

 0.000 1.750 2.250 2.388 3.700 4.000

For the normal distribution, there are functions in R to evaluate the density function, the distribution function and the quantile function (the inverse distribution function). These functions are, respectively, dnorm, pnorm, and qnorm. For example, suppose $X \sim N(3, 2^2)$; then

> dnorm(5,3,2)

will calculate the density function at point 5.

[1] 0.1209854

Note that the function assumes you will give the standard deviation rather than the variance.

As a further example

```
> x=seq(-5,5,by=.1)
> dnorm(x,3,2)
```

calculates the density function of the same distribution at intervals of 0.1 over the range [-5,5].

The functions pnorm and qnorm work in a similar way. For example, to get the probability x<4.96, you can type

```
> pnorm(4.96,3,1)
```

[1] 0.9750021

For the standard normal distribution, we can simply use

```
> pnorm(1.96)
```

[1] 0.9750021

```
> qnorm(0.975)
```

[1] 1.959964

To simulate 4 observations from the $N(1, 2^2)$ distribution we write

```
> rnorm(4,1,2)
```

[1] 0.7613512 0.3029311 3.2363236 2.5846433

Other distribution functions work similarly; you can use "Help" in R for further information.

A.2.5 *Conditional Statement and Loop*

An example of conditional statement would be

```
cat("\n","Enter x","\n") # prompt
x=scan(n=1)
2
if(x < 0){
 cat("negative")
} else{
 cat("non-negative")
}
```

It prompts you to type a value for x, the output of the result (positive or negative) dependent on your input. You try this code.

The typical loop block of statements has the form

```
for (index in 1:100) {
 #do something 100 times
}
```

or
```
for (item in a_vector) {
 #operate on item
 }
```
The line with # is the comment line. It will not be executed and there will be no effect on the program output.

A.2.6 Writing and Invoking R Function

An important feature of R is the facility to extend the language by writing your own functions. The common form for writing an R function is
```
myFunction=function ()
{
#your statements here..........
return (your value)
}
```

For example,
```
tStatistic=function(n, mu, sigma) {
x=rnorm(n, mu, sigma)
t=mean(x)/sd(x)*sqrt(n)
return (t)
}
```

This function, tStatistic, has 3 input parameters: n, mu, and sigma and an output result: t, the t-Statistic. To generate a t-Statistic for 100 observations from a normal distribution with mean (e.g., mu=0.8) and standard deviation (e.g., sigma=2), we can invoke the function using the following line of code:
```
tStatistic(100, 0.8, 2)
```
After you paste the function code and the code for invoking the function, you will get a result something like is:
```
[1] 3.338891
```
Throughout this book, we provide many functions for adaptive designs; you need to copy and paste the corresponding function for your adaptive trial simulation before you paste the invoking code. Once the function is pasted in R workspace, you can invoke it as many times as you want. You don't need to repaste the function code again unless you close the R workspace.

A.2.7 Graphics

R has many facilities for producing high-quality graphics. A useful facility before beginning is to divide a page into smaller pieces so that more than one figure can be displayed. For example:

```
> par(mfrow=c(2,2))
> x=rnorm(100,0,1)
> hist(x)
> plot(mean(x),sd(x))
> plot(x,pnorm(x))
> y=pnorm(abs(x))
> plot(x,y)
```

The lines of code will produce the graphics shown in Figure A.2.

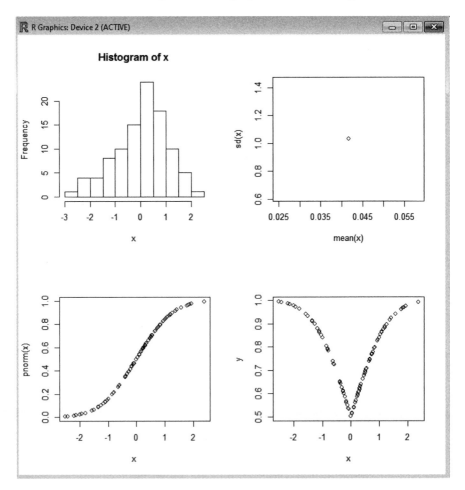

Figure A.2:   Example of R Graphics

Appendix B

R Functions for Adaptive Designs

R is a language and environment for statistical computing and graphics. It is a GNU project similar to the S language and environment which was developed at Bell Laboratories (formerly AT&T, now Lucent Technologies) by John Chambers and colleagues. R can be considered as a different implementation of S. There are some important differences, but much code written for S runs unaltered under R. R compiler is available at http://www.r-project.org/.

In this appendix, the R functions that mimic the SAS macros in each chapter are presented.

B.1 Chapter 2

```
## R Function: Dunnett Test for Multiple Arms with Common Control
    ## us[j] = true response in the jth group
    ## sigma[j] = true standard deviation for the jth group
    ## Zalpha =critical point for rejection
    ## nArms = number of active groups
    ## ns[j] = sample size for the jth group
    ## powers[j] = probability of rejection for the jth arm
    ## power = prob of at least one Hi si rejected.
    powerDunnett=function(n0, u0, sigma0, nArms, cAlpha, nSims)
    {
        powers=rep(0,nArms);      tValue=rep(0,nArms);      yCtl=rep(0,nArms);
yTest=rep(0,nArms)
    power=0

    for (i in 1: nSims) {
    yCtl=rnorm(n0, mean=u0, sd=sigma0)
    OverSig=0
    for (j in 1: nArms) {
    yTest=rnorm(ns[j],mean=us[j], sd=sigmas[j])
```

```
tValue=t.test(yTest,yCtl)$statistic
if (tValue>=cAlpha) {
powers[j]=powers[j]+1/nSims
OverSig=1}
}
power=power+OverSig/nSims
}
return (c("power=", power, "Rejection Probs = ", powers))
}
## Determine critical value Zalpha for alpha (power) =0.025 ##
ns=c(288,288,288); us=c(0,0,0); sigmas=c(2,2,2)
    powerDunnett(n0=288,    u0=0,    sigma0=2,    nArms=3,    cAlpha=2.361,
nSims=100000)


## Determine Power ##
ns=c(288,288,288); us=c(0.3,0.4,0.5); sigmas=c(2,2,2)
    powerDunnett(n0=288,    u0=0,    sigma0=2,    nArms=3,    cAlpha=2.361,
nSims=10000)
```

Examples of Invoking the Function:

```
## Determine critical value Zalpha for alpha (power) =0.025 ##
ns=c(288,288,288); us=c(0,0,0); sigmas=c(2,2,2)
    powerDunnett(n0=288,    u0=0,    sigma0=2,    nArms=3,    cAlpha=2.361,
nSims=100000)
## Determine Power ##
ns=c(288,288,288); us=c(0.3,0.4,0.5); sigmas=c(2,2,2)
    powerDunnett(n0=288,    u0=0,    sigma0=2,    nArms=3,    cAlpha=2.361,
nSims=10000)
```

B.2   Chapter 3

```
## Chapter 3-powerTwoStageClassicGSD with small or larger N
    ## sigma[j] = true standard deviation for the jth group
    ## Zalpha =critical point for rejection
    ## nArms = number of active groups
    ## ns[j] = sample size for the jth group
    ## EEP = early efficacy stopping probability
    ## power = prob of at least one Hi si rejected.
    powerTwoStageClassicGSD=function(u0,u1,sigma0,sigma1, n0Stg1, n1Stg1,
n0Stg2, n1Stg2, alpha1,beta1, alpha2, nSims)
```

```
{
power=0; EEP=0; EFP=0
for (i in 1: nSims) {
y0Stg1=rnorm(n0Stg1, mean=u0, sd=sigma0)
y1Stg1=rnorm(n1Stg1, mean=u1, sd=sigma1)
p1=t.test(y1Stg1,y0Stg1, alternative ="greater")$p.value
if(p1<=alpha1){EEP=EEP+1/nSims}
if(p1>=beta1) {EFP=EFP+1/nSims}
if(p1>alpha1 & p1<beta1) {
y0Stg2=rnorm(n0Stg2, mean=u0, sd=sigma0)
y1Stg2=rnorm(n1Stg2,mean=u1, sd=sigma1)
y0=c(y0Stg1, y0Stg2)
y1=c(y1Stg1, y1Stg2)
p2=t.test(y1,y0, alternative ="greater")$p.value
if(p2<=alpha2) {power=power+1/nSims}
}
}
power=power+EEP
aveTotalN=n0Stg1+n1Stg1+(1-EEP-EFP)*(n0Stg2+n1Stg2)
return (c("Average Total N=", aveTotalN, "power=", power, "EEP= ", EEP,
"EFP=", EFP))
}
```

Invoke the function:
Checking classic design type-I error

powerTwoStage-ClassicGSD(u0=0,u1=0,sigma0=1,sigma1=1, n0Stg1=36, n1Stg1=36, n0Stg2=36, n1Stg2=36, alpha1=0.0,beta1=1, alpha2=0.025, nSims=10000)
Checking Type-I error

powerTwoStage-ClassicGSD(u0=0,u1=0,sigma0=1,sigma1=1, n0Stg1=36, n1Stg1=36, n0Stg2=36, n1Stg2=36, alpha1=0.0024,beta1=1, alpha2=0.024, nSims=10000)
Power of Classic design

powerTwoStageClassicGSD(u0=0,u1=0.5,sigma0=1,sigma1=1, n0Stg1=36, n1Stg1=36, n0Stg2=36, n1Stg2=36, alpha1=0.0,beta1=1, alpha2=0.025, nSims=10000)
Power

powerTwoStageClassicGSD(u0=0,u1=0.5,sigma0=1,sigma1=1, n0Stg1=36, n1Stg1=36, n0Stg2=36, n1Stg2=36, alpha1=0.0024,beta1=1, alpha2=0.024, nSims=10000)

powerTwoStageClassicGSD(u0=0,u1=0.5,sigma0=1,sigma1=1, n0Stg1=58, n1Stg1=58, n0Stg2=36, n1Stg2=36, alpha1=0.025,beta1=1, alpha2=0.024, nSims=10000)

```
## Chapter 3-Two-Stage GSD of NormalEndpoint with MINP-MSP-MPP
## u0, u1 = means for two treatment groups
## sigma0, sigma1 = standard deviations for two treatment groups
## n0Stg1, n1Stg1, n0Stg2, n1Stg2 = sample sizes for the two groups at stages 1 and 2
## alpha1,beta1, alpha2 = efficacy and futility stopping boundaries
## method = adaptive design method, either MSP. MPP or MINP
## w1squared = weight squared for MINP only at stage 1
## nSims = the number of simulation runs
## ESP1, ESP2, FSP1 = efficacy and futility stopping probabilities
## power, aveTotalN = power and expected total sample size
TwoStageGSDwithNormalEndpoint=function(u0,u1,sigma0,sigma1, n0Stg1, n1Stg1, n0Stg2, n1Stg2, alpha1, beta1, alpha2, method, w1squared=0.5, nSims=100000)
{
ESP1=0; ESP2=0; FSP1=0; w1=sqrt(w1squared);
for (i in 1:nSims) {
y0Stg1=rnorm(1, u0, sigma0/sqrt(n0Stg1))
y1Stg1=rnorm(1, u1, sigma1/sqrt(n1Stg1))
z1=(y1Stg1-y0Stg1)/sqrt(sigma1**2/n1Stg1+sigma0**2/n0Stg1)
t1=1-pnorm(z1)
if(t1<=alpha1){ESP1=ESP1+1/nSims}
if(t1>=beta1) {FSP1=FSP1+1/nSims}
if(t1>alpha1 & t1<beta1) {
y0Stg2=rnorm(1, u0, sigma0/sqrt(n0Stg2))
y1Stg2=rnorm(1, u1, sigma1/sqrt(n1Stg2))
z2=(y1Stg2-y0Stg2)/sqrt(sigma1**2/n1Stg2+sigma0**2/n0Stg2)
if (method=="MINP"){t2=1-pnorm(w1*z1+sqrt(1-w1*w1)*z2)}
if (method=="MSP" ){t2=t1+pnorm(-z2)}
if (method=="MPP" ){t2=t1*pnorm(-z2)}
if(t2<=alpha2) {ESP2=ESP2+1/nSims}
}
}
power=ESP1+ESP2
aveTotalN=n0Stg1+n1Stg1+(1-ESP1-FSP1)*(n0Stg2+n1Stg2)
return (c("Average total sample size=", aveTotalN, "power=", power, "ESP1=", ESP1, "FSP1=", FSP1))
}
```

Invoke the R function:

Example 3.1

TwoStageGSDwithNormalEndpoint(u0=0.05,u1=0.12, sigma0=0.22, sigma1=0.22, n0Stg1=120, n1Stg1=120, n0Stg2=120, n1Stg2=120, alpha1=0.01, beta1=1, alpha2=0.18321, method="MSP")

TwoStageGSDwithNormalEndpoint(u0=0.05,u1=0.05, sigma0=0.22, sigma1=0.22, n0Stg1=120, n1Stg1=120, n0Stg2=120, n1Stg2=120, alpha1=0.01, beta1=1, alpha2=0.18321, method="MSP")

Example 3.2

TwoStageGSDwithNormalEndpoint(u0=0.05,u1=0.12, sigma0=0.22, sigma1=0.22, n0Stg1=113, n1Stg1=113, n0Stg2=113, n1Stg2=113, alpha1=0.01, beta1=1, alpha2=0.0033, method="MPP")

TwoStageGSDwithNormalEndpoint(u0=0.05,u1=0.05, sigma0=0.22, sigma1=0.22, n0Stg1=113, n1Stg1=113, n0Stg2=113, n1Stg2=113, alpha1=0.01, beta1=1, alpha2=0.0033, method="MPP")

Example 3.3

TwoStageGSDwithNormalEndpoint(u0=0.05,u1=0.12, sigma0=0.22, sigma1=0.22, n0Stg1=110, n1Stg1=110, n0Stg2=110, n1Stg2=110, alpha1=0.01, beta1=1, alpha2=0.0188, w1squared=0.5, method="MINP")

TwoStageGSDwithNormalEndpoint(u0=0.05,u1=0.05, sigma0=0.22, sigma1=0.22, n0Stg1=110, n1Stg1=110, n0Stg2=110, n1Stg2=110, alpha1=0.01, beta1=1, alpha2=0.0188, w1squared=0.5, method="MINP")

Example 3.4

TwoStageGSDwithNormalEndpoint(u0=0.05, u1=0.12, sigma0=0.22, sigma1=0.22, n0Stg1=124, n1Stg1=124, n0Stg2=105, n1Stg2=105, alpha1=0.0026, beta1=0.2143, alpha2=0.2143, method="MSP")

TwoStageGSDwithNormalEndpoint(u0=0.05, u1=0.05, sigma0=0.22, sigma1=0.22, n0Stg1=124, n1Stg1=124, n0Stg2=105, n1Stg2=105, alpha1=0.0026, beta1=0.2143, alpha2=0.2143, method="MSP")

TwoStageGSDwithNormalEndpoint(u0=0.05, u1=0.12, sigma0=0.22, sigma1=0.22, n0Stg1=130, n1Stg1=130, n0Stg2=105, n1Stg2=105, alpha1=0.0026, beta1=0.2143, alpha2=0.0038, method="MPP")

TwoStageGSDwithNormalEndpoint(u0=0.05, u1=0.05, sigma0=0.22, sigma1=0.22, n0Stg1=130, n1Stg1=130, n0Stg2=105, n1Stg2=105, alpha1=0.0026, beta1=0.2143, alpha2=0.0038, method="MPP")

TwoStageGSDwithNormalEndpoint(u0=0.05, u1=0.12, sigma0=0.22, sigma1=0.22, n0Stg1=116, n1Stg1=116, n0Stg2=116, n1Stg2=116, alpha1=0.0026, beta1=0.2143, alpha2=0.024, w1squared=0.5, method="MINP")

TwoStageGSDwithNormalEndpoint(u0=0.05, u1=0.05, sigma0=0.22, sigma1=0.22, n0Stg1=116, n1Stg1=116, n0Stg2=116, n1Stg2=116, alpha1=0.0026, beta1=0.2143, alpha2=0.024, w1squared=0.5, method="MINP")

Chapter 3-Two-Stage GSD of Various Endpoints with MINP-MSP-MPP
Two-Stage GSD for Different Endpoints with MINP, MSP, and MPP
u0, u1 = true means of the group
NId = noninferiority margin
sigma0, sigma1 = standard deviation for groups 0 and 1
nStg1, nStg2 = sample sizes per group at stages 1 and 2
alpha1, beta1, alpha2 = stopping boundaries for the two stages
tStd, tAcr = study and accrual durations
endpoint = normal, binary, or survival
method = MINP, MSP, or MPP
tStd, tAcr = time of study and time of accrual for survival study
u0, u1 = means, proportions, or hazard rates for the two groups
w1quared = the weight w1-squared at stage 1 of MINP
ESP1, ESP2, FSP1 = efficacy and futility stopping probability at stages 1 and 2
power, aveN = power and average sample size per group
number of simulation runs

```
TwoStageGSDwithVariousEndpoints=function(u0,u1,sigma0=1,  sigma1=1,
tStd=24, tAcr=9, nStg1, nStg2, alpha1, beta1=0.5, alpha2, method="MINP", end-
point="normal", NId=0, w1squared=0.5, nSims=100000)
{
w1=sqrt(w1squared); w2=sqrt(1-w1squared)
if (endpoint=="binary") {sigma0=sqrt(u0*(1-u0)); sigma1=sqrt(u1*(1-u1))}
if (endpoint=="survival") {
Expu0d=exp(-u0*tStd); Expu1d=exp(-u1*tStd);
sigma0=u0*(1+Expu0d*(1-exp(u0*tAcr))/(tAcr*u0))**(-0.5);
sigma1=u1*(1+Expu1d*(1-exp(u1*tAcr))/(tAcr*u1))**(-0.5);
}
aveN=0; ESP1=0; ESP2=0; FSP1=0
for (i in 1:nSims) {
y0Stg1=rnorm(1, u0, sigma0/sqrt(nStg1))
y1Stg1=rnorm(1, u1, sigma1/sqrt(nStg1))
z1=(y1Stg1-y0Stg1+NId)/sqrt(sigma1**2/nStg1+sigma0**2/nStg1)
t1=1-pnorm(z1)
if(t1<=alpha1){ESP1=ESP1+1/nSims}
if(t1>=beta1) {FSP1=FSP1+1/nSims}
aveN=aveN+nStg1/nSims
if(t1>alpha1 & t1<beta1) {
y0Stg2=rnorm(1, u0, sigma0/sqrt(nStg2))
y1Stg2=rnorm(1, u1, sigma1/sqrt(nStg2))
z2=(y1Stg2-y0Stg2+NId)/sqrt(sigma1**2/nStg2+sigma0**2/nStg2)
if (method=="MINP"){t2=1-pnorm(w1*z1+w2*z2)}
```

```
if (method=="MSP" ){t2=t1+pnorm(-z2)}
if (method=="MPP" ){t2=t1*pnorm(-z2)}
if(t2<=alpha2) {ESP2=ESP2+1/nSims}
aveN=aveN+nStg2/nSims
}
}
power=ESP1+ESP2
return (c("Average n per group=", aveN, "power=", power, "ESP1= ", ESP1,
"FSP1=", FSP1))
}
```

Invoke the function:

Example 3.5

```
                                                              TwoStageGSD-
withVariousEndpoints(u0=0.12,u1=0.14, nStg1=2580, nStg2=2580, alpha1=0.0026,
beta1=0.5, alpha2=0.024, method="MINP", w1squared=0.5, endpoint="binary")
                                                              TwoStageGSD-
withVariousEndpoints(u0=0.14,u1=0.14, nStg1=2580, nStg2=2580, alpha1=0.0026,
beta1=0.5, alpha2=0.024, method="MINP", w1squared=0.5, endpoint="binary")
```

Example 3.6

```
          TwoStageGSDwithVariousEndpoints(u0=0.06601,          u1=0.08664,
nStg1=190, nStg2=190, alpha1=0.0026, beta1=1, alpha2=0.024, method="MINP",
w1squared=0.5, endpoint="survival")
          TwoStageGSDwithVariousEndpoints(u0=0.08664,          u1=0.08664,
nStg1=190, nStg2=190, alpha1=0.0026, beta1=1, alpha2=0.024, method="MINP",
w1squared=0.5, endpoint="survival")
```

Example 3.7

```
          TwoStageGSDwithVariousEndpoints(u0=0.06601,          u1=0.08664,
nStg1=123, nStg2=123, alpha1=0.0026, beta1=1, alpha2=0.024, method="MINP",
w1squared=0.5, endpoint="survival", NId=0.005)
          TwoStageGSDwithVariousEndpoints(u0=0.08664+0.005,    u1=0.08664,
nStg1=123, nStg2=123, alpha1=0.0026, beta1=1, alpha2=0.024, method="MINP",
w1squared=0.5, endpoint="survival", NId=0.005)
```

Chapter 3-Two-Stage GSD for Different Endpoints with MINP-MSP-MPP for Superiority and NI Trial

```
## Two-Stage SSR for Different Endpoints with MINP, MSP, and MPP
## sigma0, sigma1 = standard deviation for groups 0 and 1
## nStg1 = sample size per group at stage 1
## alpha1, beta1, alpha2 = stopping boundaries for the two stages
## tStd, tAcr = study and accrual durations
## endpoint = normal, binary, or survival
```

power = prob of at least one Hi si rejected.
method = MINP, MSP, or MPP
tStd, tAcr = time of study and time of acrural for survuval study
u0, u1 = means, proportions, or hazard rates for the two groups
w1quared = the weight w1-squared at stage 1 of MINP
NId = noninferiority margin, NId=0 for superiority design
ESP1, ESP2, FSP1 = efficacy and futility stopping probability at stages 1 and 2
power, aveN = power and average sample size per group
number of simulation runs

```
TwoStageGSDwithVariousEndpoints=function(u0,u1,sigma0=1, sigma1=1,
tStd=24, tAcr=9, nStg1, nStg2, alpha1, beta1, alpha2, method, end-
point="normal", w1squared=0.5, NId=0, nSims=100000)
{
w1=sqrt(w1squared); w2=sqrt(1-w1squared)
if (endpoint=="binary") {sigma0=sqrt(u0*(1-u0)); sigma1=sqrt(u1*(1-u1))}
if (endpoint=="survival") {
Expu0d=exp(-u0*tStd); Expu1d=exp(-u1*tStd);
sigma0=u0*(1+Expu0d*(1-exp(u0*tAcr))/(tAcr*u0))**(-0.5);
sigma1=u1*(1+Expu1d*(1-exp(u1*tAcr))/(tAcr*u1))**(-0.5);
}
aveN=0; ESP1=0; ESP2=0; FSP1=0 ; u1=u1+NId
for (i in 1:nSims) {
y0Stg1=rnorm(1, u0, sigma0/sqrt(nStg1))
y1Stg1=rnorm(1, u1, sigma1/sqrt(nStg1))
z1=(y1Stg1-y0Stg1)/sqrt(sigma1**2/nStg1+sigma0**2/nStg1)
t1=1-pnorm(z1)
if(t1<=alpha1){ESP1=ESP1+1/nSims}
if(t1>=beta1) {FSP1=FSP1+1/nSims}
aveN=aveN+nStg1/nSims
if(t1>alpha1 & t1<beta1) {
y0Stg2=rnorm(1, u0, sigma0/sqrt(nStg2))
y1Stg2=rnorm(1, u1, sigma1/sqrt(nStg2))
z2=(y1Stg2-y0Stg2)/sqrt(sigma1**2/nStg2+sigma0**2/nStg2)
if (method=="MINP"){t2=1-pnorm(w1*z1+w2*z2)}
if (method=="MSP" ){t2=t1+pnorm(-z2)}
if (method=="MPP" ){t2=t1*pnorm(-z2)}
if(t2<=alpha2) {ESP2=ESP2+1/nSims}
aveN=aveN+nStg2/nSims
}
}
power=ESP1+ESP2
```

return (c("Average N per group=", aveN, "power=", power, "ESP1= ", ESP1, "FSP1=", FSP1))
}

Invoke the function:
Example 3.5

TwoStageGSD-withVariousEndpoints(u0=0.12,u1=0.14, nStg1=2580, nStg2=2580, alpha1=0.0026, beta1=0.5, alpha2=0.024, method="MINP", w1squared=0.5, endpoint="binary")

TwoStageGSD-withVariousEndpoints(u0=0.14,u1=0.14, nStg1=2580, nStg2=2580, alpha1=0.0026, beta1=0.5, alpha2=0.024, method="MINP", w1squared=0.5, endpoint="binary")

Example 3.6

TwoStageGSDwithVariousEndpoints(u0=0.06601, u1=0.08664, nStg1=190, nStg2=190, alpha1=0.0026, beta1=1, alpha2=0.024, method="MINP", w1squared=0.5, endpoint="survival")

TwoStageGSDwithVariousEndpoints(u0=0.08664, u1=0.08664, nStg1=190, nStg2=190, alpha1=0.0026, beta1=1, alpha2=0.024, method="MINP", w1squared=0.5, endpoint="survival")

Example 3.7

TwoStageGSDwithVariousEndpoints(u0=0.06601, u1=0.08664, nStg1=123, nStg2=123, alpha1=0.0026, beta1=1, alpha2=0.024, method="MINP", w1squared=0.5, endpoint="survival", NId=0.005)

TwoStageGSDwithVariousEndpoints(u0=0.08664+0.005, u1=0.08664, nStg1=123, nStg2=123, alpha1=0.0026, beta1=1, alpha2=0.024, method="MINP", w1squared=0.5, endpoint="survival", NId=0.005)

B.3   Chapter 4

Chapter 4-K-Stage Group-Sequential DesignwithMINP for NormalEndpoint
    ## ux, uy = true treatment means for groups x and y
    ## sigmax, sigmay = true standard deviation for groups x and y
    ## alphas = efficacy stopping boundaries
    ## betas = efficacy stopping boundaries
    ## Nx[i],Ny[i] = subsample size at stage i for groups x and y
    ## ESP = efficacy stopping probability
    ## FSP = efficacy stopping probability
    ## nStgs = number of stages of the trial
    ## w[k,i] = weights, calculated based on info time
    ## power, aveN = power and the average total sample size
    TwoArmKStgGSDwithMINPNormalEndpoint = function (nSims=100000, nStgs=2, ux=0, uy=1, NId=0, sigmax=1,sigmay=1) {

```
AveTotalN=0; FSP=rep(0, nStgs); ESP=rep(0, nStgs); sumWs=rep(0, nStgs)
w=matrix(rep(0,nStgs), nrow=nStgs, ncol=nStgs, byrow = TRUE)
for (k in 1:nStgs) {
for (i in 1:k) {sumWs[k]=sumWs[k]+(Nx[i]+Ny[i])**2}
sumWs[k]=sqrt(sumWs[k])
}
for (k in 1:nStgs){for (i in 1:k){w[k,i]=(Nx[i]+Ny[i])/sumWs[k]}}
for (iSim in 1:nSims) {
TS=0; TSc=rep(0, nStgs)
for (i in 1:nStgs) {
uxObs=rnorm(1, ux, sigmax/sqrt(Nx[i]))
uyObs=rnorm(1, uy, sigmay/sqrt(Ny[i]))
TS0=(uyObs-uxObs+NId)/sqrt(sigmax**2/Nx[i]+sigmay**2/Ny[i])
for (k in 1:nStgs) {TSc[k]=TSc[k]+w[k,i]*TS0}
TS=1-pnorm(TSc[i])
AveTotalN=AveTotalN+(Nx[i]+Ny[i])/nSims
if (TS<=alphas[i]){ESP[i]=ESP[i]+1/nSims; break}
if (TS>betas[i]) { FSP[i]=FSP[i]+1/nSims; break}
} # End of i
} # End of iSim
power=0; for (i in 1:nStgs) {power=power+ESP[i]}
return (c("power=", power, "Average total N =", AveTotalN, "ESP=", ESP,
"FSP=", FSP))
}
```

Invoke the function:

```
# Example 4.4: Three-Stage Design
Nx = c(92,92,92); Ny = c(92,92,92); alphas = c(0.0025, 0.00575, 0.022); betas
= c(0.5, 0.5, 0.022)
TwoArmKStgGSDwithMINPNormalEndpoint(nSims=100000, nStgs=3, ux=0,
uy=0, NId=0, sigmax=0.22, sigmay=0.22)
TwoArmKStgGSDwithMINPNormalEndpoint(nSims=100000,      nStgs=3,
ux=0.05, uy=0.12, NId=0, sigmax=0.22, sigmay=0.22)
TwoArmKStgGSDwithMINPNormalEndpoint(nSims=100000,      nStgs=3,
ux=0.05, uy=0.10, NId=0, sigmax=0.22, sigmay=0.22)
## Chapter 4-K-Stage GSD for Different Endpoints with MINP-MSP-MPP for
Superiority and NI Trial
## ux, uy = means, proportions, or hazard rates for the two groups
## sigmax, sigmay = true standard deviation for groups x and y
## alphas = efficacy stopping boundaries
## betas = efficacy stopping boundaries
## Nx[i],Ny[i] = subsample size at stage i for groups x and y
```

```
## ESP = efficacy stopping probability
## FSP = efficacy stopping probability
## nStgs = number of stages of the trial
## w[k,i] = weights, calculated based on info time
## power, aveN = power and the average total sample size
## endpoint = normal, binary, or survival
## method = MINP, MSP, or MPP
## tStd, tAcr = time of study and time of accrual for survival study


KStgGSDwithVariousEndpointsForMspMppMinp=function (ux=0.2, uy=0.3,
sigmax=1, sigmay=1, tStd=24, tAcr=9, nStgs=3, method="MINP", end-
point="normal", NId=0, nSims=10000)
{
w=matrix(rep(0,nStgs), nrow=nStgs, ncol=nStgs, byrow = TRUE)
sumWs=rep(0, nStgs)
for (k in 1:nStgs) {
for (i in 1:k) {sumWs[k]=sumWs[k]+(Nx[i]+Ny[i])**2}
sumWs[k]=sqrt(sumWs[k])
}
## Determine the equivalent std dev.
if (endpoint=="binary") {
sigmax=sqrt(ux*(1-ux));
sigmay=sqrt(uy*(1-uy))+0.000000001} # to avoid numerical overflow
if (endpoint=="survival") {
Expuxd=exp(-ux*tStd); Expuyd=exp(-uy*tStd);
sigmax=ux*(1+Expuxd*(1-exp(ux*tAcr))/(tAcr*ux))**(-0.5);
sigmay=uy*(1+Expuyd*(1-exp(uy*tAcr))/(tAcr*uy))**(-0.5);
}
for (k in 1:nStgs){for (i in 1:k){w[k,i]=(Nx[i]+Ny[i])/sumWs[k]}}
AveTotalN=0; FSP=rep(0, nStgs); ESP=rep(0, nStgs); uy=uy+NId

for (iSim in 1:nSims) {
TS=0; TSc=rep(0, nStgs); if (method=="MPP") {TSc=rep(1, nStgs)}
for (i in 1:nStgs) {
uxObs=rnorm(1, ux, sigmax/sqrt(Nx[i]))
uyObs=rnorm(1, uy, sigmay/sqrt(Ny[i]))
TS0=(uyObs-uxObs+NId)/sqrt(sigmax**2/Nx[i]+sigmay**2/Ny[i])
for (k in 1:nStgs) {
if (method=="MINP") {TSc[k]=TSc[k]+w[k,i]*TS0}
if (method=="MSP") {TSc[k]=TSc[k]+pnorm(-TS0)}
if (method=="MPP") {TSc[k]=TSc[k]*pnorm(-TS0)}
}
```

```
if (method=="MINP") {TSc[i]=pnorm(-TSc[i])} ## Convert to p-scale
AveTotalN=AveTotalN+(Nx[i]+Ny[i])/nSims
if (TSc[i]<=alphas[i]){ESP[i]=ESP[i]+1/nSims; break}
if (TSc[i]>betas[i]) { FSP[i]=FSP[i]+1/nSims; break}
} # End of i
} # End of iSim
power=0; for (i in 1:nStgs) {power=power+ESP[i]}
return (c("power=", power, "Average total N =", AveTotalN, "ESP=", ESP,
"FSP=", FSP))
}
```

Invoke the function:

```
# Example 4.4: Three-Stage Design Normal endpoint
Nx = c(92,92,92); Ny = c(92,92,92); alphas = c(0.0025, 0.00575, 0.022); betas
= c(0.5, 0.5, 0.022)
    KStgGSDwithVariousEndpointsForMspMppMinp(ux=0,     uy=0,     sig-
max=0.22, sigmay=0.22, nStgs=3, method="MINP", endpoint="normal", NId=0,
nSims=10000)
    KStgGSDwithVariousEndpointsForMspMppMinp(ux=0.05,  uy=0.12,  sig-
max=0.22, sigmay=0.22, nStgs=3, method="MINP", endpoint="normal", NId=0,
nSims=10000)
    KStgGSDwithVariousEndpointsForMspMppMinp(ux=0.05,  uy=0.1,   sig-
max=0.22, sigmay=0.22, nStgs=3, method="MINP", endpoint="normal", NId=0,
nSims=10000)
Nx = c(92,92,92); Ny = c(92,92,92); alphas = c(0.0025, 0.1025, 0.49257); betas
= c(0.49257, 0.49257, 0.49257)
    KStgGSDwithVariousEndpointsForMspMppMinp(ux=0,     uy=0,     sig-
max=0.22, sigmay=0.22, nStgs=3, method="MSP", endpoint="normal", NId=0,
nSims=10000)
    KStgGSDwithVariousEndpointsForMspMppMinp(ux=0.05,  uy=0.12,  sig-
max=0.22, sigmay=0.22, nStgs=3, method="MSP", endpoint="normal", NId=0,
nSims=10000)
    KStgGSDwithVariousEndpointsForMspMppMinp(ux=0.05,  uy=0.10,  sig-
max=0.22, sigmay=0.22, nStgs=3, method="MSP", endpoint="normal", NId=0,
nSims=10000)

# Example 4.5: Three-Stage Design binary endpoint
Nx = c(1860,1860,1860); Ny = c(1860,1860,1860); alphas = c(0.005, 0.00653,
0.0198); betas = c(0.45, 0.45, 0.0198)
                                                             KStgGSD-
withVariousEndpointsForMspMppMinp(ux=0, uy=0, nStgs=3, method="MINP",
endpoint="binary", NId=0, nSims=10000)
```

KStgGSDwithVariousEndpointsForMspMppMinp(ux=0.12, uy=0.14, nStgs=3, method="MINP", endpoint="binary", NId=0, nSims=10000)

Nx = c(1860,1860,1860); Ny = c(1860,1860,1860); alphas = c(0.0025, 0.00083452, 0.00071363); betas = c(1,1,0.00071363)

KStgGSDwithVariousEndpointsForMspMppMinp(ux=0, uy=0, nStgs=3, method="MPP", endpoint="binary", NId=0, nSims=10000)

KStgGSDwithVariousEndpointsForMspMppMinp(ux=0.12, uy=0.14, nStgs=3, method="MPP", endpoint="binary", NId=0, nSims=10000)

B.4   Chapter 5

```
## Chapter 5-Two-Stage MaxInfo Design for Normal Endpoint
    ## Sample Size Reestimation with the Mixed Method
    ## SSR Design with Small or Larger Sample Size
    ## sigma[j] = true standard deviation for the jth group
    ## alpha1, alpha2, beta1 = stopping boundaries on p-scale
    ## u0, u1 = true means for the two groups
    ## delta0 = estimated mean difference u1-u0
    ## nStg1, nStg2 = sample sizes for stage 1 and 2
    ## Nmin, Nmax = minimum and maximum sample sizes allowed for SSR
    ## ESP1, ESP2, FSP = efficacy and futility stopping probabilities
    ## aveN = average sample size per group
    TwoStageMaxInfoSSRDesign=function(u0,u1,sigma0,sigma1, delta0, nStg1,
Nmin=72, Nmax=200, alpha=0.025, cPower=0.9, nSims=10000)
    {
    ESP1=0; ESP2=0; FSP1=0; aveN=0; nFinal=Nmin
    for (i in 1: nSims) {
    y0Stg1=rnorm(nStg1, u0, sigma0)
    y1Stg1=rnorm(nStg1, u1, sigma1)
    p1=t.test(y1Stg1,y0Stg1, alternative ="greater")$p.value
    aveN=aveN+nStg1/nSims
    ## New n2 by mixed method
    yStg1=c(y0Stg1, y1Stg1)
    sigmaBlind=sd(yStg1)
    if (sigmaBlind>0) {
                        nFinal=2*((sigmaBlind/delta0)**2-1/4)*(qnorm(1-
alpha)+qnorm(cPower))**2-nStg1
    ## Force Nmin<=nFinal<=Nmax
    nFinal=round(min(max(nFinal,Nmin),Nmax))
    }
```

```
nStg2=nFinal-nStg1; aveN=aveN+nStg2/nSims
y0Stg2=rnorm(nStg2, u0, sigma0)
y1Stg2=rnorm(nStg2, u1, sigma1)
y0=c(y0Stg1, y0Stg2); y1=c(y1Stg1, y1Stg2)
p2=t.test(y1,y0, alternative ="greater")$p.value
if(p2<=alpha) {ESP2=ESP2+1/nSims}
}
power=ESP1+ESP2
return (c(sigmaBlind, nFinal, "Power=", power, "Average N=", aveN, "ESP1=
", ESP1, "FSP1=", FSP1))
}
```

Invoke the function:

Checking classic design type-I error

```
                                              TwoStageMaxInfoS-
SRDesign(u0=0,u1=0,sigma0=3,sigma1=3, delta0=0.3, nStg1=1050, Nmin=2100,
Nmax=4000, alpha=0.025, cPower=0.9)
```

Power of MaxInfo SSR design

```
TwoStageMaxInfoSSRDesign(u0=0,u1=.25,sigma0=3,sigma1=3,  delta0=0.3,
nStg1=1050, Nmin=2100, Nmax=4000, alpha=0.025, cPower=0.9)
TwoStageMaxInfoSSRDesign(u0=0,u1=.30,sigma0=3,sigma1=3,  delta0=0.3,
nStg1=1050, Nmin=2100, Nmax=4000, alpha=0.025, cPower=0.9)
TwoStageMaxInfoSSRDesign(u0=0,u1=.30,sigma0=4,sigma1=4,  delta0=0.3,
nStg1=1050, Nmin=2100, Nmax=4000, alpha=0.025, cPower=0.9)
TwoStageMaxInfoSSRDesign(u0=0,u1=.35,sigma0=3,sigma1=3,  delta0=0.3,
nStg1=1050, Nmin=2100, Nmax=4000, alpha=0.025, cPower=0.9)
```

```
## Chapter 5-Two-Stage Unblind SSR for Normal Endpoints with MINP-MSP-
MPP
## u0 and u1 = parameter means for the two groups
## sigma = common standard deviation
## alpha1, alpha2, beta1 = stopping boundaries on p-scale
## nStg1, nStg2 = sample size for stages 1 and 2
## nMax = maximum sample size per group
## w1= stage-1 weight in MINP only
## ESP = efficacy stopping probability
## FSP = futility stopping probability
## power = prob of rejecting Ha.
## NId = noninferiority margin
## cPower = the targeted conditional power
## n2 = new sample size per group for stage 2
## aveN = average sample size per group
```

method = MINP, MSP, or MPP

```
                                    powerTwoStageUnblindSSRnormal-
Endpoint=function(u0,u1,sigma, nStg1, nStg2, alpha1,beta1=0.205, alpha2,NId=0,
cPower, method, nMax=100, w1=0.7071, nSims=100000)
   {
   power=0; aveN=0; ESP=0; FSP=0; w2=sqrt(1-w1**2); n2=nStg2
   for (i in 1: nSims) {
   y0Stg1=rnorm(1, mean=u0, sd=sigma/sqrt(nStg1))
   y1Stg1=rnorm(1, mean=u1, sd=sigma/sqrt(nStg1))
   z1=(y1Stg1-y0Stg1)/sigma*sqrt(nStg1/2)
   t1=1-pnorm(z1)
   aveN=aveN+nStg1/nSims
   if(t1<=alpha1){ESP=ESP+1/nSims}
   if(t1>=beta1) {FSP=FSP+1/nSims}
   if(t1>alpha1 & t1<beta1) {
   # n2 by conditional power
   if (method=="MSP") {BFun = qnorm(1-max(0.00001,alpha2-t1))}
   if (method=="MPP") {BFun = qnorm(1- min(0.99999,alpha2/t1))}
   if (method=="MINP"){BFun = (qnorm(1-alpha2)- w1*qnorm(1-t1))/w2}
   eSize=(y1Stg1-y0Stg1+NId)/sigma
                if        (eSize        >0)            {n2=min(nMax-nStg1,
max(2*((BFun-qnorm(1-cPower))/eSize)**2, nStg2))}

   y0Stg2=rnorm(1, mean=u0, sd=sigma/sqrt(n2))
   y1Stg2=rnorm(1, mean=u1, sd=sigma/sqrt(n2))
   z2=(y1Stg2-y0Stg2)/sigma*sqrt(n2/2)

   if (method=="MSP" ){t2=t1+pnorm(-z2)}
   if (method=="MPP" ){t2=t1*pnorm(-z2)}
   if (method=="MINP"){t2=1-pnorm(w1*z1+w2*z2)}
   if(t2<=alpha2) {power=power+1/nSims}
   aveN=aveN+n2/nSims
   }
   } # End of iSim
   power=power+ESP
   return (c("Average N=", aveN, "power=", power, "ESP= ", ESP, "FSP=",
FSP))
   }
```

Invoke the function:
Example 5.1
Checking Type-I error with MINP

powerTwoStageUnblindSSRnormal-
Endpoint(u0=0,u1=0,sigma=1, nStg1=80, nStg2=80, alpha1=0.0026, beta1=0.205,
alpha2=0.024, cPower=0.9, method="MINP", nMax=320, w1=0.7071)
Power with MINP under Ha

powerTwoStageUnblindSSRnormalEnd-
point(u0=0,u1=0.33,sigma=1, nStg1=80, nStg2=80, alpha1=0.0026, beta1=0.205,
alpha2=0.024, cPower=0.9, method="MINP", nMax=320, w1=0.7071)
Power with MINP under Hs

powerTwoStageUnblindSSRnormalEnd-
point(u0=0,u1=0.28,sigma=1, nStg1=80, nStg2=80, alpha1=0.0026, beta1=0.205,
alpha2=0.024, cPower=0.9, method="MINP", nMax=320, w1=0.7071)
# Checking Type-I error with MSP ##

powerTwoStageUnblindSSRnormalEndpoint(u0=0,u1=0,sigma=1,
nStg1=80, nStg2=80, alpha1=0.0026, beta1=0.205, alpha2=0.21463, cPower=0.9,
method="MSP", nMax=320)
Power with MSP under Ha

powerTwoStageUnblindSSRnormalEndpoint(u0=0,u1=0.33,sigma=1,
nStg1=80, nStg2=80, alpha1=0.0026, beta1=0.205, alpha2=0.21463, cPower=0.9,
method="MSP", nMax=320)
Power with MSP under Hs

powerTwoStageUnblindSSRnormalEndpoint(u0=0,u1=0.28,sigma=1,
nStg1=80, nStg2=80, alpha1=0.0026, beta1=0.205, alpha2=0.21463, cPower=0.9,
method="MSP", nMax=320)
Checking Type-I error with MPP##

powerTwoStageUnblindSSRnormal-
Endpoint(u0=0,u1=0,sigma=1, nStg1=80, nStg2=80, alpha1=0.0025, beta1=0.205,
alpha2=0.0038, cPower=0.9, method="MPP",nMax=320)
Power with MPP##

powerTwoStageUnblindSSRnormalEnd-
point(u0=0,u1=0.33,sigma=1,nStg1=80, nStg2=80, alpha1=0.0025, beta1=0.205,
alpha2=0.0038, cPower=0.9, method="MPP",nMax=320)
Power with MPP##

powerTwoStageUnblindSSRnormalEnd-
point(u0=0,u1=0.28,sigma=1,nStg1=80, nStg2=80, alpha1=0.0025, beta1=0.205,
alpha2=0.0038, cPower=0.9, method="MPP",nMax=320)
# Table 5.4
# Checking Type-I error with MINP ##
powerTwoStageUnblindSSRnormalEndpoint(u0=0,u1=0,sigma=3, nStg1=800,
nStg2=800, alpha1=0, beta1=0.5, alpha2=0.025, cPower=0.9, method="MINP",
nMax=4000, w1=0.7071)

powerTwoStageUnblindSSRnormal-
Endpoint(u0=0,u1=0.25,sigma=3, nStg1=800, nStg2=800, alpha1=0, beta1=0.5,

alpha2=0.025, cPower=0.9, method="MINP", nMax=3000, w1=0.7071)

powerTwoStageUnblindSSRnormal-
Endpoint(u0=0,u1=0.30,sigma=3, nStg1=800, nStg2=800, alpha1=0, beta1=0.5,
alpha2=0.025, cPower=0.9, method="MINP", nMax=3000, w1=0.7071)

powerTwoStageUnblindSSRnormal-
Endpoint(u0=0,u1=0.30,sigma=4, nStg1=800, nStg2=800, alpha1=0, beta1=0.5,
alpha2=0.025, cPower=0.9, method="MINP", nMax=3000, w1=0.7071)

powerTwoStageUnblindSSRnormal-
Endpoint(u0=0,u1=0.35,sigma=3, nStg1=800, nStg2=800, alpha1=0, beta1=0.5,
alpha2=0.025, cPower=0.9, method="MINP", nMax=3000, w1=0.7071)

Chapter 5-Two-Stage Unblind SSR for Different Endpoints with MINP-MSP-MPP

Two-Stage SSR for Different Endpoints with MINP, MSP, and MPP

sigma0, sigma1 = standard deviation for groups 0 and 1

nStg1 = sample size per group at stage 1

alpha1, beta1, alpha2 = stopping boundaries for the two stages

tStd, tAcr = study and accrual durations

endpoint = normal, binary, or survival

power = prob of at least one Hi si rejected.

method = MINP, MSP, or MPP

tStd, tAcr = time of study and time of accrual for survival study

u0, u1 = means, proportions, or hazard rates for the two groups

w1quared = the weight w1-squared at stage 1 of MINP

Nmin, Nmax = minimum and maximum sample size per group allowed in SSR

cPower = the targeted conditional power in SSR

ESP1, ESP2, FSP1 = efficacy and futility stopping probability at stages 1 and 2

power, aveN = power and average sample size per group

number of simulation runs

TwoStageSS-
RwithVariousEndpoints=function(u0,u1,sigma0=1, sigma1=1, tStd=24, tAcr=9,
nStg1, alpha1, beta1=0.5, alpha2, method="MINP", endpoint="normal", NId=0,
w1squared=0.5, Nmin, Nmax, cPower=0.9, nSims=100000)

```
{
w1=sqrt(w1squared); w2=sqrt(1-w1squared); n2=Nmin-nStg1
if (endpoint=="binary") {sigma0=sqrt(u0*(1-u0)); sigma1=sqrt(u1*(1-u1))}
if (endpoint=="survival") {
Expu0d=exp(-u0*tStd); Expu1d=exp(-u1*tStd);
sigma0=u0*(1+Expu0d*(1-exp(u0*tAcr))/(tAcr*u0))**(-0.5)
sigma1=u1*(1+Expu1d*(1-exp(u1*tAcr))/(tAcr*u1))**(-0.5)
}
```

```
        sigma=sqrt(sigma0**2+sigma1**2)
        aveN=0; ESP1=0; ESP2=0; FSP1=0
        for (i in 1:nSims) {
        y0Stg1=rnorm(1, u0, sigma0/sqrt(nStg1))
        y1Stg1=rnorm(1, u1, sigma1/sqrt(nStg1))
        z1=(y1Stg1-y0Stg1+NId)/sqrt(sigma1**2/nStg1+sigma0**2/nStg1)
        t1=1-pnorm(z1)
        if(t1<=alpha1){ESP1=ESP1+1/nSims}
        if(t1>=beta1) {FSP1=FSP1+1/nSims}
        aveN=aveN+nStg1/nSims
        if(t1>alpha1 & t1<beta1) {
        # new n2 by conditional power
        if (method=="MSP") {BFun=qnorm(1-max(0.000001,alpha2-t1))}
        if (method=="MPP") {BFun=qnorm(1- min(0.999999,alpha2/t1))}
        if (method=="MINP"){BFun=(qnorm(1-alpha2)- w1*qnorm(1-t1))/w2}
        eSize=(y1Stg1-y0Stg1+NId)/sigma
            n2=round(min(Nmax-nStg1,      max(2*((BFun-qnorm(1-cPower))/eSize)^2,
Nmin-nStg1)))
        y0Stg2=rnorm(1, u0, sigma0/sqrt(n2))
        y1Stg2=rnorm(1, u1, sigma1/sqrt(n2))
        z2=(y1Stg2-y0Stg2+NId)/sqrt(sigma1**2/n2+sigma0**2/n2)
        if (method=="MINP"){t2=1-pnorm(w1*z1+w2*z2)}
        if (method=="MSP" ){t2=t1+pnorm(-z2)}
        if (method=="MPP" ){t2=t1*pnorm(-z2)}
        if(t2<=alpha2) {ESP2=ESP2+1/nSims}
        aveN=aveN+n2/nSims
        }
        }
        power=ESP1+ESP2
        return (c("Average n per group=", aveN, "power=", power, "ESP1= ", ESP1,
"FSP1=", FSP1))
        }
```

Invoke the function:

```
## Example 5.2
## Classic design
    TwoStageSSRwithVariousEndpoints(u0=0.22,u1=0.22, nStg1=145, alpha1=0,
beta=1, alpha2=0.025, method="MINP", endpoint="binary", w1squared=0.5,
Nmin=290, Nmax=290, nSims=100000)
    TwoStageSSRwithVariousEndpoints(u0=0.10,u1=0.22, nStg1=145, alpha1=0,
beta=1, alpha2=0.025, method="MINP", endpoint="binary", w1squared=0.5,
Nmin=290, Nmax=290, nSims=100000)
```

TwoStageSSRwithVariousEndpoints(u0=0.11,u1=0.22, nStg1=145, alpha1=0, beta=1, alpha2=0.025, method="MINP", endpoint="binary", w1squared=0.5, Nmin=290, Nmax=290, nSims=100000)

TwoStageSSRwithVariousEndpoints(u0=0.14,u1=0.22, nStg1=145, alpha1=0, beta=1, alpha2=0.025, method="MINP", endpoint="binary", w1squared=0.5, Nmin=290, Nmax=290, nSims=100000)

GSD with OBF boundary

TwoStageSSRwithVariousEndpoints(u0=0.22,u1=0.22, nStg1=150, alpha1=0.0026, beta=0.5, alpha2=0.024, method="MINP", endpoint="binary", w1squared=0.5, Nmin=300, Nmax=300, cPower=0.9, nSims=100000)

TwoStageSSRwithVariousEndpoints(u0=0.10,u1=0.22, nStg1=150, alpha1=0.0026, beta=0.5, alpha2=0.024, method="MINP", endpoint="binary", w1squared=0.5, Nmin=300, Nmax=300, cPower=0.9, nSims=100000)

TwoStageSSRwithVariousEndpoints(u0=0.11,u1=0.22, nStg1=150, alpha1=0.0026, beta=0.5, alpha2=0.024, method="MINP", endpoint="binary", w1squared=0.5, Nmin=300, Nmax=300, cPower=0.9, nSims=100000)

TwoStageSSRwithVariousEndpoints(u0=0.14,u1=0.22, nStg1=150, alpha1=0.0026, beta=0.5, alpha2=0.024, method="MINP", endpoint="binary", w1squared=0.5, Nmin=300, Nmax=300, cPower=0.9, nSims=100000)

SSR Design with OBF boundary

TwoStageSSRwithVariousEndpoints(u0=0.22,u1=0.22, nStg1=100, alpha1=0.0026, beta=0.5, alpha2=0.024, method="MINP", endpoint="binary", w1squared=0.5, Nmin=180, Nmax=410, cPower=0.9, nSims=100000)

TwoStageSSRwithVariousEndpoints(u0=0.10,u1=0.22, nStg1=100, alpha1=0.0026, beta=0.5, alpha2=0.024, method="MINP", endpoint="binary", w1squared=0.5, Nmin=180, Nmax=410, cPower=0.9, nSims=100000)

TwoStageSSRwithVariousEndpoints(u0=0.11,u1=0.22, nStg1=100, alpha1=0.0026, beta=0.5, alpha2=0.024, method="MINP", endpoint="binary", w1squared=0.5, Nmin=180, Nmax=410, cPower=0.9, nSims=100000)

TwoStageSSRwithVariousEndpoints(u0=0.14,u1=0.22, nStg1=100, alpha1=0.0026, beta=0.5, alpha2=0.024, method="MINP", endpoint="binary", w1squared=0.5, Nmin=180, Nmax=410, cPower=0.9, nSims=100000)

```
## Chapter 5-Two-Stage Mixed SSR Design with Normal Endpoint
## Sample Size Reestimation with the Mixed Method
## SSR Design with Small or Larger Sample Size
## sigma[j] = true standard deviation for the jth group
## alpha1, alpha2, beta1 = stopping boundaries on p-scale
## u0, u1 = true means for the two groups
## delta0 = estimated mean difference u1-u0
## nStg1, nStg2 = sample sizes for stage 1 and 2
## Nmin, Nmax = minimum and maximum sample sizes allowed for SSR
## ESP1, ESP2, FSP = efficacy and futility stopping probabilities
## aveN = average sample size per group
TwoStageMixedSSRDesignWithNormalEndpoint=function(u0,u1,sigma0,sigma1, delta0, nStg1, Nmin=72, Nmax=200, alpha1,beta1, alpha2, cPower=0.9, nSims=10000)
{
ESP1=0; ESP2=0; FSP1=0; aveN=0; nFinal=Nmin
for (i in 1: nSims) {
y0Stg1=rnorm(nStg1, u0, sigma0)
y1Stg1=rnorm(nStg1, u1, sigma1)
p1=t.test(y1Stg1,y0Stg1, alternative ="greater")$p.value
aveN=aveN+nStg1/nSims
if(p1<=alpha1){ESP1=ESP1+1/nSims}
if(p1>=beta1) {FSP1=FSP1+1/nSims}
if(p1>alpha1 & p1<beta1) {
## New n2 by mixed method
yStg1=c(y0Stg1, y1Stg1)
sigmaBlind=sd(yStg1)
if (sigmaBlind>0) {
eSize=delta0/sigmaBlind
BFun=sqrt(2)*qnorm(1-alpha2)-qnorm(1-p1);
nFinal=nStg1+2*((BFun-qnorm(1-cPower))/eSize)**2
## Force Nmin<=nFinal<=Nmax
nFinal=round(min(max(nFinal,Nmin),Nmax))
}
nStg2=nFinal-nStg1; aveN=aveN+nStg2/nSims
y0Stg2=rnorm(nStg2, u0, sigma0)
y1Stg2=rnorm(nStg2, u1, sigma1)
y0=c(y0Stg1, y0Stg2); y1=c(y1Stg1, y1Stg2)
p2=t.test(y1,y0, alternative ="greater")$p.value
if(p2<=alpha2) {ESP2=ESP2+1/nSims}
}
}
```

power=ESP1+ESP2

return (c("Power=", power, "Average N=", aveN, "ESP1= ", ESP1, "FSP1=", FSP1))

}

Invoke the function:

Table 5.4

Checking Mixed SRR design type-I error

TwoStageMixedSSRDesignWithNormal-Endpoint(u0=0,u1=0,sigma0=3,sigma1=3, delta0=0.3, nStg1=900, Nmin=1800, Nmax=4000, alpha1=0,beta1=0.5, alpha2=0.025, cPower=0.9, nSims=100000)

Power of Classic design

TwoStageMixedSSRDesignWithNormal-Endpoint(u0=0,u1=0.25,sigma0=3,sigma1=3, delta0=0.3, nStg1=900, Nmin=1800, Nmax=4000, alpha1=0,beta1=0.5, alpha2=0.025, cPower=0.9, nSims=10000)

TwoStageMixedSSRDesignWithNormal-Endpoint(u0=0,u1=0.3,sigma0=3,sigma1=3, delta0=0.3, nStg1=900, Nmin=1800, Nmax=4000, alpha1=0,beta1=0.5, alpha2=0.025, cPower=0.9, nSims=10000)

TwoStageMixedSSRDesignWithNormal-Endpoint(u0=0,u1=0.3,sigma0=4,sigma1=4, delta0=0.3, nStg1=900, Nmin=1800, Nmax=4000, alpha1=0,beta1=0.5, alpha2=0.025, cPower=0.9, nSims=10000)

TwoStageMixedSSRDesignWithNormal-Endpoint(u0=0,u1=0.35,sigma0=3,sigma1=3, delta0=0.3, nStg1=900, Nmin=1800, Nmax=4000, alpha1=0,beta1=0.5, alpha2=0.025, cPower=0.9, nSims=10000)

Chapter 5-Two-Stage Mixed and Unblind SSR Design with Binary Endpoint

Two-Stage SSR for Binary Endpoint with Mixed and Unblinded MINP

nStg1 = sample size per group at stage 1

alpha1, beta1, alpha2 = stopping boundaries for the two stages

power = prob of at least one Hi si rejected.

px, py = proportions for the two groups

Nmin, Nmax = minimum and maximum sample size per group allowed in SSR

cPower = the targeted conditional power in SSR

ESP1, ESP2, FSP1 = efficacy and futility stopping probability at stages 1 and 2

power, aveN = power and average sample size per group

number of simulation runs

TwoStageMixedSSRwithBinaryEndpoint=function(px, py, nStg1, alpha1, beta1=0.5, alpha2, px0=0.11, py0=0.22, NId=0, SSR="mixed", Nmin, Nmax, cPower=0.9, nSims=100000)

```
{
w1=sqrt(nStg1/Nmin); w2=sqrt(1-w1*w1); n2=Nmin-nStg1

aveN=0; ESP1=0; ESP2=0; FSP1=0
for (i in 1:nSims) {
pxStg1=rbinom(1, nStg1, px)/nStg1
pyStg1=rbinom(1, nStg1, py)/nStg1
sigma=sqrt(pxStg1*(1-pxStg1)+pyStg1*(1-pyStg1))
sigmaBlind=sqrt(2*(pxStg1+pyStg1)/2*(1-(pxStg1+pyStg1)/2))
z1=(pyStg1-pxStg1+NId)/sqrt(sigma**2/nStg1)
t1=1-pnorm(z1)
if(t1<=alpha1){ESP1=ESP1+1/nSims}
if(t1>=beta1) {FSP1=FSP1+1/nSims}
aveN=aveN+nStg1/nSims
if(t1>alpha1 & t1<beta1) {
# new n2 by conditional power
BFun=(qnorm(1-alpha2)- w1*qnorm(1-t1))/w2
if (SSR=="unblind"){eSize=(pyStg1-pxStg1+NId)/sigma}
if (SSR=="mixed"){eSize=(py0-px0+NId)/sigmaBlind}
   n2=round(min(Nmax-nStg1,   max(2*((BFun-qnorm(1-cPower))/eSize)**2,
Nmin-nStg1)))
pxStg2=rbinom(1, n2, px)/n2
pyStg2=rbinom(1, n2, py)/n2
sigma=sqrt(pxStg2*(1-pxStg2)+pyStg2*(1-pyStg2))
z2=(pyStg2-pxStg2+NId)/sqrt(sigma**2/n2)
t2=1-pnorm(w1*z1+w2*z2)
if(t2<=alpha2) {ESP2=ESP2+1/nSims}
aveN=aveN+n2/nSims
}
}
power=ESP1+ESP2
return (c("Average n per group=", aveN, "power=", power, "ESP1= ", ESP1,
"FSP1=", FSP1))
}
```

Invoke the function:
```
## Example 5.2
## Classic design
   TwoStageMixedSSRwithBinaryEndpoint(px=0.22,py=0.22, nStg1=145, al-
pha1=0, beta=1, alpha2=0.025, SSR="unblind", Nmin=290, Nmax=290,
nSims=100000)

   TwoStageMixedSSRwithBinaryEndpoint(px=0.10,py=0.22, nStg1=145, al-
```

pha1=0, beta=1, alpha2=0.025, SSR="unblind", Nmin=290, Nmax=290, nSims=100000)

TwoStageMixedSSRwithBinaryEndpoint(px=0.11,py=0.22, nStg1=145, alpha1=0, beta=1, alpha2=0.025, SSR="unblind", Nmin=290, Nmax=290, nSims=100000)

TwoStageMixedSSRwithBinaryEndpoint(px=0.14,py=0.22, nStg1=145, alpha1=0, beta=1, alpha2=0.025, SSR="unblind", Nmin=290, Nmax=290, nSims=100000)

GSD with OBF boundary

TwoStageMixedSSRwithBinaryEndpoint(px=0.22,py=0.22, nStg1=150, alpha1=0.0026, beta=0.5, alpha2=0.024, SSR="unblind", Nmin=300, Nmax=300, cPower=0.9, nSims=100000)

TwoStageMixedSSRwithBinaryEndpoint(px=0.10,py=0.22, nStg1=150, alpha1=0.0026, beta=0.5, alpha2=0.024, SSR="unblind", Nmin=300, Nmax=300, cPower=0.9, nSims=100000)

TwoStageMixedSSRwithBinaryEndpoint(px=0.11,py=0.22, nStg1=150, alpha1=0.0026, beta=0.5, alpha2=0.024, SSR="unblind", Nmin=300, Nmax=300, cPower=0.9, nSims=100000)

TwoStageMixedSSRwithBinaryEndpoint(px=0.14,py=0.22, nStg1=150, alpha1=0.0026, beta=0.5, alpha2=0.024, SSR="unblind", Nmin=300, Nmax=300, cPower=0.9, nSims=100000)

Unblind SSR Design with OBF boundary

TwoStageMixedSSRwithBinaryEndpoint(px=0.22,py=0.22, nStg1=100, alpha1=0.0026, beta=0.5, alpha2=0.024, SSR="unblind", Nmin=200, Nmax=410, cPower=0.9, nSims=100000)

TwoStageMixedSSRwithBinaryEndpoint(px=0.10,py=0.22, nStg1=100, alpha1=0.0026, beta=0.5, alpha2=0.024, SSR="unblind", Nmin=200, Nmax=410, cPower=0.9, nSims=100000)

TwoStageMixedSSRwithBinaryEndpoint(px=0.11,py=0.22, nStg1=100, alpha1=0.0026, beta=0.5, alpha2=0.024, SSR="unblind", Nmin=200, Nmax=410, cPower=0.9, nSims=100000)

TwoStageMixedSSRwithBinaryEndpoint(px=0.14,py=0.22, nStg1=100, alpha1=0.0026, beta=0.5, alpha2=0.024, SSR="unblind", Nmin=200, Nmax=410, cPower=0.9, nSims=100000)

Mixed SSR Design with OBF boundary

TwoStageMixedSSRwithBinaryEndpoint(px=0.22,py=0.22, nStg1=100, alpha1=0.0026, beta=0.5, alpha2=0.024, SSR="mixed", Nmin=200, Nmax=410, cPower=0.9, nSims=100000)

TwoStageMixedSSRwithBinaryEndpoint(px=0.10,py=0.22, nStg1=100, alpha1=0.0026, beta=0.5, alpha2=0.024, SSR="mixed", Nmin=200, Nmax=410, cPower=0.9, nSims=100000)

TwoStageMixedSSRwithBinaryEndpoint(px=0.11,py=0.22, nStg1=100, alpha1=0.0026, beta=0.5, alpha2=0.024, SSR="mixed", Nmin=200, Nmax=410, cPower=0.9, nSims=100000)

TwoStageMixedSSRwithBinaryEndpoint(px=0.14,py=0.22, nStg1=100, alpha1=0.0026, beta=0.5, alpha2=0.024, SSR="mixed", Nmin=200, Nmax=410, cPower=0.9, nSims=100000)

GSD with OBF boundary

TwoStageMixedSSRwithBinaryEndpoint(px=0.22,py=0.22, nStg1=200, alpha1=0.0026, beta=0.5, alpha2=0.024, SSR="unblind", Nmin=400, Nmax=400, cPower=0.9, nSims=100000)

TwoStageMixedSSRwithBinaryEndpoint(px=0.10,py=0.22, nStg1=200, alpha1=0.0026, beta=0.5, alpha2=0.024, SSR="unblind", Nmin=400, Nmax=400, cPower=0.9, nSims=100000)

TwoStageMixedSSRwithBinaryEndpoint(px=0.11,py=0.22, nStg1=200, alpha1=0.0026, beta=0.5, alpha2=0.024, SSR="unblind", Nmin=400, Nmax=400, cPower=0.9, nSims=100000)

TwoStageMixedSSRwithBinaryEndpoint(px=0.14,py=0.22, nStg1=200, alpha1=0.0026, beta=0.5, alpha2=0.024, SSR="unblind", Nmin=400, Nmax=400, cPower=0.9, nSims=100000)

B.5   Chapter 6

Chapter 6-ADwithIncompletePairs

ADwithIncompletePairs=function(alpha=0.025, alpha1=0.00153, alpha2=0.02454, beta1=1, sigma=0.433, NewSigma=0.489, N1=100, N2=100, Nmin=200, Nmax=250, u=0.1, cPower=0.9, nSims=100000)
{
w1=sqrt(N1/(N1+N2)); w2=sqrt(1-w1**2); FSP1=0; ESP1=0; ESP2=0; aveN=0;
for (iSim in 1:nSims) {
uObs=rnorm(1, u, sigma/sqrt(N1))
z1=uObs*sqrt(N1)/sigma
p1=1-pnorm(z1)
aveN=aveN+N1/nSims
if (p1>beta1){FSP1=FSP1+1/nSims}
if (p1<=alpha1){ESP1=ESP1+1/nSims}
if (p1>alpha1 & p1<=beta1){
nFinal=2*((NewSigma/u)**2-1/4)*(qnorm(1-alpha)+qnorm(cPower))**2
nFinal=round(min(max(nFinal,Nmin),Nmax))
NewN2=nFinal-N1

```
z2=rnorm(1,u*sqrt(NewN2)/NewSigma,1)
TS2=w1*z1+w2*z2; p2=1-pnorm(TS2);
if (p2<=alpha2) {ESP2=ESP2+1/nSims}
aveN=aveN+NewN2/nSims
}
} ## End of iSim
Power = ESP1+ESP2
return (c("power=", Power, "Average N=", aveN, "ESP1=", ESP1, "FSP1=",
FSP1))
}
```

Invoke the function
```
## Classical under Ha Power
    ADwithIncompletePairs(alpha=0.025,  alpha1=.025,  alpha2=0,  beta1=0.5,
sigma=0.433, NewSigma=0.433, N1=200, N2=0, Nmax = 200, u=0.1, cPower=0.9,)
    ADwithIncompletePairs(alpha=0.025,  alpha1=.025,  alpha2=0,  beta1=0.5,
sigma=0.489, NewSigma=0.489, N1=200, N2=0, Nmax = 200, u=0.1, cPower=0.9,)
    ## Two-stage Adaptive Design with Blind SSR
    ADwithIncompletePairs(alpha=0.025,    alpha1=0.0026,    alpha2=0.024,
beta1=0.5, sigma=0.433, NewSigma=0.489, N1=100, N2=100, Nmin=200, Nmax
= 250, u=0.1, cPower=0.9)


## Chapter 6-GSDwithCoprimaryEndpoints
## Two-group, two-endpoint with two stage design
## muij= standardized means of j endpoint in group i
## rho= the true correlation between the two endpoints
## c1 and c2 = stopping boundaries
## N= maximum sample size per group
## tau = info time for the interim analysis
library(mvtnorm)
        GSDwithCoprimaryEndpoints=function(mu11,mu12,          mu21,
mu22,rho,tau,c1,c2,N,nSims=10000)
{
ESP1=0; ESP2=0
for (i in 1:nSims)
{
n=round(N*tau)
varcov=matrix(c(1,rho,rho,1),2,2)
trtStg1=rmvnorm(n,mean=c(mu11,mu12), sigma=varcov)
ctStg1 =rmvnorm(n,mean=c(mu21,mu22),sigma=varcov)
t11=t.test(trtStg1[,1],ctStg1[,1])$statistic
t12=t.test(trtStg1[,2],ctStg1[,2])$statistic
```

```
trtStg2=rmvnorm(N-n, mean=c(mu11,mu12), sigma=varcov)
ctStg2 =rmvnorm(N-n, mean=c(mu21,mu22), sigma=varcov)
trt1=c(trtStg1[,1],trtStg2[,1]); trt2=c(trtStg1[,2],trtStg2[,2])
ct1 =c(ctStg1[,1] ,ctStg2[,1]); ct2 =c(ctStg1[,2] ,ctStg2[,2])
t21=t.test(trt1,ct1)$statistic; t22=t.test(trt2,ct2)$statistic
## if ((t11>c1 & t12>c1) | (t21>c2 & t22>c2)) {power=power+1/nSims}
if (t11>c1 & t12>c1){ESP1=ESP1+1/nSims}
else {if (t21>c2 & t22>c2){ESP2=ESP2+1/nSims}}
power=ESP1+ESP2; aveN=n+(1-ESP1)*(N-n)
}
return (c("Power=", power, "Average N=", aveN))
}
```

Invoke the function:

```
GSDwithCoprimaryEndpoints(mu11=0.2,mu12=0.25,            mu21=0.005,
mu22=0.015, rho=0.25, tau=0.5, c1=2.80, c2=1.98, N=584, nSims=10000)
      GSDwithCoprimaryEndpoints(mu11=0.5,mu12=0.5, mu21=0, mu22=0, rho=0,
tau=0.5, c1=2.80, c2=1.98, N=84, nSims=10000)
      GSDwithCoprimaryEndpoints(mu11=0.5,mu12=0.5, mu21=0, mu22=0, rho=1,
tau=0.5, c1=2.80, c2=1.98, N=84, nSims=10000)
```

```
## Chapter 6-NIADwithPairedBinaryData
## Adaptive Noninferiority Design with Paired Binary Data */
## Ho: p10-p01-delNI <= 0 */
## p10 and p01 are the % of disconcordant pairs */
## Sample size: nPairs = nPairs1 + nPairs2 from stage 1 and 2 */
## avenPairs = the expected sample size (pairs)
## alpha = one-sided significance level
## ESP1, ESP2 = rejection probability at stages 1 and 2
## FSP1 = acceptance probability at stage 1
## alpha1, alpha2=, beta1 = stopping boundaries on p-scale
## nPairsMax = max number of pairs, TargetcPow=targeted conditional power
## w1 = the first stage weight, w2=sqrt(1-w1**2)
## delNI = the noninferiority margin
      McNemarADwithSSR=function(alpha1=0.0026,            alpha2=0.024,
beta1=1, p10=0.125, p01=0.125, delNI=0.1, nPairs1=154, nPairs2=154, nPairs-
Max=600, TargetcPow=0.90, w1=0.707, nSims=10000)
  {
      w2=sqrt(1-w1**2);    ESP1=0;    ESP2=0;    FSP1=0;    avenPairs=0;
nPairs20=nPairs2
    for (iSim in 1:nSims) {
    avenPairs=avenPairs+nPairs1/nSims
```

```
n10Stg1=rbinom(1, nPairs1,p10); n01Stg1=rbinom(1,nPairs1,p01)
p10obsStg1=n10Stg1/nPairs1; p01obsStg1=n01Stg1/nPairs1
epsStg1=p10obsStg1-p01obsStg1-delNI
b=(2+p01obsStg1-p10obsStg1)*delNI-p01obsStg1-p10obsStg1
c=-p01obsStg1*delNI*(1-delNI)
p01Wave=(-b+sqrt(b*b-8*c))/4
sigma2Stg1=2*p01Wave+delNI-delNI**2
z1=0; if (sigma2Stg1 != 0) {z1=epsStg1*sqrt(nPairs1/sigma2Stg1)}
pValue1=1-pnorm(z1); t1=pValue1
if (t1<=alpha1) {ESP1=ESP1+1/nSims}
if (t1>beta1) {FSP1=FSP1+1/nSims}
if (alpha1<t1 & t1<=beta1) {
## Sample size reestimation based on conditional power
Bval=(qnorm(1-alpha2)-w1*z1)/w2
nPairs2=nPairs20
if (epsStg1>0) {
nPairs2=sigma2Stg1/epsStg1**2*(Bval-qnorm(1-TargetcPow))**2
nPairs2=min(nPairsMax-nPairs1,nPairs2)
nPairs2=round(max(nPairs2, nPairs20))
} ## End of SSR
n10Stg2=rbinom(1,nPairs2,p10); n01Stg2=rbinom(1,nPairs2,p01)
p10obsStg2=n10Stg2/nPairs2; p01obsStg2=n01Stg2/nPairs2
epsStg2=p10obsStg2-p01obsStg2-delNI
b=(2+p01obsStg2-p10obsStg2)*delNI-p01obsStg2-p10obsStg2
c=-p01obsStg2*delNI*(1-delNI);
p01Wave=(-b+sqrt(b*b-8*c))/4;
sigma2Stg2=2*p01Wave+delNI-delNI**2;
z2=0; if (sigma2Stg2 !=0) {z2=epsStg2*sqrt(nPairs2/sigma2Stg2)}
pValue2=1-pnorm(z2); t2=1-pnorm(w1*z1+w2*z2)
if (t2<=alpha2) ESP2=ESP2+1/nSims
avenPairs=avenPairs+nPairs2/nSims;
} # End of Stage 2
} # End of isim
Power=ESP1+ESP2
 return (c("Power=", Power, "Average N=", avenPairs, "ESP1=", ESP1,
"ESP2=", ESP2, "FSP1=", FSP1))
 }
```

Invoke the function:

```
## Classical 1-Stage Design : Type-I error rate p10-p01-delNI=0
McNemarADwithSSR(alpha1=0.025, alpha2=0, beta1=0, p10=0.1, p01=0.175,
delNI=-0.075, nPairs1=322, nPairs2=0);
```

```
## Power for design with PF (rho=2), beta1=0.5 and SSR (Nmax>N0)
McNemarADwithSSR(alpha1=0.00625, alpha2=0.02173, beta1=0.5, p10=0.1,
p01=0.1, delNI=-0.075, nPairs1=161, nPairs2=161, nPairsMax=500);


## Chapter 6-Two Stage Farrington-Manning NI Trial with SSR
## u0 and u1 = parameter means for the two groups
## sigma = common standard deviation
## alpha1, alpha2, beta1 = stopping boundaries on p-scale
## nStg1, nStg2 = sample size for stages 1 and 2
## nMax = maximum sample size per group
## w1= stage-1 weight in MINP only
## ESP = efficacy stopping probability
## FSP = futility stopping probability
## power = prob of rejecting Ha.
## NId = NI margin, NId=0.1 means retain 90% effect size
## cPower = the targeted conditional power
## n2 = new sample size per group for stage 2
## aveN = average sample size per group
## method = MINP, MSP, or MPP
                                          powerTwoStageFarringtonManningNI-
withSSRnormalEndpoint=function(u0,u1,sigma, nStg1, nStg2, alpha1,beta1=0.205,
alpha2,NId=0.1, cPower, method, nMax=100, w1=0.7071, nSims=100000)
    {
    power=0; aveN=0; ESP=0; FSP=0; w2=sqrt(1-w1**2); n2=nStg2
    for (i in 1: nSims) {
    y0Stg1=rnorm(1, mean=u0, sd=sigma/sqrt(nStg1))
    y1Stg1=rnorm(1, mean=u1, sd=sigma/sqrt(nStg1))
    z1=(y1Stg1-(1-NId)*y0Stg1)/sigma*sqrt(nStg1/(2-NId))
    t1=1-pnorm(z1)
    aveN=aveN+nStg1/nSims
    if(t1<=alpha1){ESP=ESP+1/nSims}
    if(t1>=beta1) {FSP=FSP+1/nSims}
    if(t1>alpha1 & t1<beta1) {
    # n2 by conditional power
    BFun = (qnorm(1-alpha2)- w1*qnorm(1-t1))/w2
    eSize=(y1Stg1-y0Stg1+NId)/sigma
           if         (eSize         >0)          {n2=min(nMax-nStg1,
max(2*((BFun-qnorm(1-cPower))/eSize)**2, nStg2))}

    y0Stg2=rnorm(1, mean=u0, sd=sigma/sqrt(n2))
    y1Stg2=rnorm(1, mean=u1, sd=sigma/sqrt(n2))
    z2=(y1Stg2-(1-NId)*y0Stg2)/sigma*sqrt(n2/(2-NId))
```

```
t2=1-pnorm(w1*z1+w2*z2)
if(t2<=alpha2) {power=power+1/nSims}
aveN=aveN+n2/nSims
}
} # End of iSim
power=power+ESP
return (c("Average N=", aveN, "power=", power, "ESP= ", ESP, "FSP=",
FSP))
}
```

Invoke the function:

```
# Example 6.2: Adaptive Design with Farrington-Manning NI Margin
                                                 powerTwoStageFarring-
tonManningNIwithSSRnormalEndpoint(u0=0.20,u1=0.20,sigma=0.08, nStg1=150,
nStg2=150, alpha1=0.0026, beta1=0.205, alpha2=0.024, NId=0.1, cPower=0.9,
method="MINP", nMax=320, w1=0.7071)
```

```
## Chapter 6-Two-Stage Equivalence GSD of NormalEndpoint MINP
## du = mean difference between the two treatment groups
## sigma = common standard deviations
## nStg1, nStg2 = sample sizes per group at stages 1 and 2
## alpha1,beta1, alpha2 = efficacy and futility stopping boundaries
## w1squared = weight squared for MINP only at stage 1
## nSims = the number of simulation runs
## ESP1, ESP2, FSP1 = efficacy and futility stopping probabilities
## power, aveN = power and expected sample size per group
    TwoStageEquivGSDwithNormalEndpoint=function(du,sigma, Eqd, nStg1,
nStg2, alpha1, beta1, alpha2, w1squared=0.5, nSims=100000)
{
ESP1=0; ESP2=0; FSP1=0; w1=sqrt(w1squared); w2=sqrt(1-w1*w1)
for (i in 1:nSims) {
dyStg1=rnorm(1, du, sigma/sqrt(nStg1/2))
z1=(Eqd-abs(dyStg1))/sigma*sqrt(nStg1/2)
t1=1-pnorm(z1)
if(t1<=alpha1){ESP1=ESP1+1/nSims}
if(t1>=beta1) {FSP1=FSP1+1/nSims}
if(t1>alpha1 & t1<beta1) {
dyStg2=rnorm(1, du, sigma/sqrt(nStg2/2))
z2=(Eqd-abs(dyStg2))/sigma*sqrt(nStg2/2)
t2=1-pnorm(w1*z1+w2*z2)
if(t2<=alpha2) {ESP2=ESP2+1/nSims}
}
```

```
}
power=ESP1+ESP2
aveN=nStg1+(1-ESP1-FSP1)*nStg2
return (c("Average N per group=", aveN, "power=", power, "ESP1= ", ESP1,
"FSP1=", FSP1))
}
```

Invoke the function:

Example 6.1: Type I error control with O'Brien-Fleming Boundary is conservative since the pdf of the test statistics has heavy tails.

TwoStageEquivGSDwithNormalEndpoint(du=0.2, sigma=0.72, Eqd=0.2, nStg1=200, nStg2=200, alpha1=0.0052, beta1=1, alpha2=0.048, w1squared=0.5, nSims=1000000)

Example 6.1: Power GSD for Equivalence Trial

TwoStageEquivGSDwithNormalEndpoint(du=0, sigma=0.72, Eqd=0.2, nStg1=200, nStg2=200, alpha1=0.0052, beta1=1, alpha2=0.048, w1squared=0.5, nSims=100000)

Example 6.1: Type I error control

TwoStageEquivGSDwithNormalEndpoint(du=0.2, sigma=0.72, Eqd=0.2, nStg1=200, nStg2=200, alpha1=0.0085, beta1=1, alpha2=0.048, w1squared=0.5, nSims=1000000)

Example 6.1: Power GSD for Equivalence Trial

TwoStageEquivGSDwithNormalEndpoint(du=0, sigma=0.72, Eqd=0.2, nStg1=200, nStg2=200, alpha1=0.0085, beta1=1, alpha2=0.048, w1squared=0.5, nSims=100000)

B.6   Chapter 7

Chapter 7-Classic K+1 Drop-Arm Design

```
## The Classical ACTIVE K+1 Arm dropping-Loser Design
## Large sample size assumption
## H0: all means are equal. Ha: at least one mean > mean0.
## For Dunnett's test, nStage2=0.
WinnerDesign=function(nSims=1000,NumOfArms=5, mu0=0, sigma=1,
Z_alpha=2.407, nStg1=100, nStg2=100){
xObs=rep(0,NumOfArms); power=0
for (iSim in 1:nSims) {
for (i in 1:NumOfArms){xObs[i]=rnorm(1,mu[i],sigma/sqrt(nStg1))}
MaxRsp =xObs[1]; SelectedArm=1
for (i in 1:NumOfArms) {
if (xObs[i]> MaxRsp) {SelectedArm=i; MaxRsp=xObs[i]}
```

```
}
x2=rnorm(1,mu[SelectedArm],sigma/max(1,sqrt(nStg2)))
FinalxAve=(MaxRsp*nStg1+x2*nStg2)/(nStg1+nStg2)
x0Ave=rnorm(1,mu0,sigma/sqrt(nStg1+nStg2))
TestZ=(FinalxAve-x0Ave)*sqrt((nStg1+nStg2)/2)/sigma
if (TestZ >= Z_alpha){power=power+1/nSims}
}
TotalN=(NumOfArms+1)*nStg1+2*nStg2
return (c("Power=", power, "Total N=", TotalN))
}
```

Invoke the function:

```
## Determine Critical Value Z_alpha for 4+1 Arms Winner Design
mu=c(0,0,0,0)
```

```
WinnerDesign(nSims=1000000,NumOfArms=4, mu0=0, sigma=1, Z_alpha=2.352,
nStg1=60, nStg2=60)
```

```
## Determine Power for 4+1 Arms Winner Design
mu=c(0.12, 0.13, 0.14, 0.15)
     WinnerDesign(nSims=100000,NumOfArms=4,      mu0=0.06,      sigma=0.18,
Z_alpha=2.352, nStg1=60, nStg2=60)
```

```
## Determine Critical Value Z_alpha for 4+1 Arms Winner Design
mu=c(0,0,0,0)
     WinnerDesign(nSims=1000000,NumOfArms=4,       mu0=0,       sigma=1,
Z_alpha=2.3, nStg1=43, nStg2=86)
```

```
## Determine Power for 4+1 Arms Winner Design
mu=c(0.12, 0.13, 0.14, 0.15)
     WinnerDesign(nSims=100000,NumOfArms=4,      mu0=0.06,      sigma=0.18,
Z_alpha=2.3, nStg1=43, nStg2=86)
```

```
## Determine Critical Value Z_alpha for Dunnett Test
mu=c(0,0,0,0)
```

```
WinnerDesign(nSims=1000000,NumOfArms=4, mu0=0, sigma=1, Z_alpha=2.441,
nStg1=102, nStg2=0);
```

```
## Determine Power for Dunnett Test
mu=c(0.12, 0.13, 0.14, 0.15);
     WinnerDesign(nSims=100000,NumOfArms=4,      mu0=0.06,      sigma=0.18,
Z_alpha=2.441, nStg1=102, nStg2=0)
```

B.7   Chapter 8

```
## Chapter 8-FourPlusOneAddArmDesign
   ##SelProb[i] = probability of selecting arm i as the best arm
   FourPlus1AddArmDesign=function(nSims=10000, N1=100, N2=100, c_alpha
= 2.267,cR = 0.55652, mu0=0, sigma=1)
   {
   Power=0; SelProb=rep(0,4); xObs=rep(0,4)
   for (iSim in 1:nSims){
   for (i in 1:4){xObs[i]=rnorm(1,mu[i],sigma/sqrt(N1))}
   if (xObs[2]>xObs[3]){
   SelectedArm=2
   if (xObs[1]*sqrt(N1)/sigma>xObs[2]*sqrt(N1)/sigma-cR) {SelectedArm=1}
   }
   if (xObs[2]<=xObs[3]){
   SelectedArm=3
   if (xObs[4]*sqrt(N1)/sigma>xObs[3]*sqrt(N1)/sigma-cR) {SelectedArm=4}
   }
   MaxRsp = xObs[SelectedArm]
   x2=rnorm(1,mu[SelectedArm], sigma/sqrt(N2))
   FinalxAve = (MaxRsp*N1+x2*N2)/(N1+N2)
   x0Ave = rnorm(1,mu0,sigma/sqrt(N1+N2))
   TestZ=(FinalxAve-x0Ave)*sqrt((N1+N2)/2)/sigma
   if (TestZ >= c_alpha) {Power=Power+1/nSims}
   for (i in 1:4){if (SelectedArm==i){SelProb[i]=SelProb[i]+1/nSims}}
   } #End of iSim
   TotalN=4*N1+2*N2
   return (c("power=", Power, "Sample Size=", TotalN, "Selection Prob=", Sel-
Prob))
   }
```

Invoke the function:

```
   mu=c(0,0,0,0)
   FourPlus1AddArmDesign(nSims=100000,  N1=100,  N2=100,  c_alpha =
2.267,cR = 0.55652, mu0=0, sigma=1)
   mu=c(0.4,0.58,0.7,0.45)
   FourPlus1AddArmDesign(nSims=10000, N1=116, N2=116, c_alpha = 2.267,cR
= 0.55652, mu0=0.35, sigma=0.9)
   mu=c(0,0,0,0)
   FourPlus1AddArmDesign(nSims=100000, N1=30, N2=70, c_alpha = 2.267,cR
= 0.55652, mu0=0, sigma=1)
```

B.8   Chapter 9

Chapter 9-BiomarkerEnrichmentDesign
   ## mup, mun = treatment effects for biomarker positive and negative populations
   ## sigma = common standard deviation for treatment effect
   ## Np1, Np2, Nn1, Nn2 = sample size for biomarker positive and negative at stages 1 and 2
   ## c_alpha = critical value for rejection
   ## powerP, powerO, power = powers for biomarker positive, negative, and either of them

```
      BiomarkerEnrichmentDesign=function(nSims=10000,mup=0.5,     mun=0,
sigma=1, Np1=100, Np2=100, Nn1=100, Nn2=100, c_alpha = 2.2)
   {
      Np=Np1+Np2;     Nn=Nn1+Nn2;     TotalN=Np+Nn;     N1=Np1+Nn1;
N2=Np2+Nn2
      power=0; powerO=0; powerP=0; aveN=0
      for (iSim in 1:nSims){
      xp1=rnorm(1,mup,sigma/sqrt(Np1))
      xn1=rnorm(1,mun,sigma/sqrt(Nn1))
      x1=(xp1*Np1+xn1*Nn1)/N1
      tp1=xp1*sqrt(Np1)/sigma
      t1=x1*sqrt(N1)/sigma
      xp2=rnorm(1,mup,sigma/sqrt(Np2))
      xn2=rnorm(1,mun,sigma/sqrt(Nn2))
      x2=(xp2*Np2+xn2*Nn2)/N2
      tp2=xp2*sqrt(Np2)/sigma
      t2=x2*sqrt(Np)/sigma
      tp=sqrt(Np1/Np)*tp1+sqrt(Np2/Np)*tp2
      t=sqrt(Np1/N1)*t1+sqrt(Np2/N2)*t2
      aveN=aveN+(Np1+Np2+Nn1+Nn2)/nSims
      if (tp1>t1) aveN=aveN-Nn2/nSims
      if (tp1>t1 & tp>c_alpha) {powerP=powerP+1/nSims}
      if (tp1<=t1 & t>c_alpha) {powerO=powerO+1/nSims}
      if ((tp1>t1 & tp>c_alpha)|(tp1<=t1 & t>c_alpha)) {power=power+1/nSims}
      } #End of iSim
      return (c("Average N=", aveN, "power=", power, "powerP=", powerP,
"powerO=", powerO))
   }
```

   Invoke the function:
   # # Simulation of Global H0 Design 1 (Nn1=Nn2=200)

BiomarkerEnrichmentDesign(nSims=1000000,mup=0,   mun=0,   sigma=1.2,
Np1=200, Np2=200, Nn1=200, Nn2=200, c_alpha = 2.13)

Simulation of Ha: Design 1 (Nn1=Nn2=200)

BiomarkerEnrichmentDesign(nSims=100000,mup=0.2, mun=0.05, sigma=1.2,
Np1=200, Np2=200, Nn1=200, Nn2=200, c_alpha = 2.13)

Simulation of Global H0 Design 2 (Nn1=Nn2=105)

BiomarkerEnrichmentDesign(nSims=1000000,mup=0,   mun=0,   sigma=1.2,
Np1=210, Np2=210, Nn1=105, Nn2=105, c_alpha = 2.39)

Simulation of H: Design 2 (Nn1=Nn2=105)

BiomarkerEnrichmentDesign(nSims=100000,mup=0.2, mun=0.05, sigma=1.2,
Np1=210, Np2=210, Nn1=105, Nn2=105, c_alpha = 2.39)

```
## Chapter 9-Biomarker-Informed Design with Hierarchical Model
## R-Function 9.2: Biomarker-Informed Design with Hierarchical Model
## u0y[j], u0x[j], rhou, suy sux = parameters of the parent model in group j
## rho, sy, sx = parameters in the lower level model
## Zalpha =critical point for rejection
## nArms = number of active groups
## N1 and N = sample size per group at interim and final analyses
## probWinners = probability of selecting the arm as the winner
library(mvtnorm)
powerBInfo=function(uCtl, u0y, u0x, rhou, suy, sux ,rho, sy, sx, Zalpha, N1, N,
nArms, nSims)
{
uy=rep(0,nArms); ux=rep(0,nArms); probWinners=rep(0,nArms); power = 0
varcov0=matrix(c(suy^2,rhou*suy*sux,rhou*suy*sux, sux^2),2,2)
varcov=matrix(c(sy^2, rho*sy*sx, rho*sx*sy, sx^2),2,2)
for (i in 1: nSims) {
winnerMarker= -Inf
for (j in 1: nArms) {
u=rmvnorm(1,mean=c(u0y[j],u0x[j]), sigma=varcov0)
uy[j]=u[1]; ux[j]=u[2]
dataStg1=rmvnorm(N1, mean=c(uy[j], ux[j]), sigma=varcov)
meanxMarker=mean(dataStg1[,2])
if (meanxMarker>winnerMarker)
{winner=j; winnerMarker=meanxMarker; winnerY=dataStg1[,1]}
} ## End of j ##
for (j in 1:nArms) {if (winner==j) {probWinners[j]=probWinners[j]+1/nSims}}
yStg1=winnerY
yStg2=rnorm(N-N1, mean=uy[winner], sd=sy)
yTrt=c(yStg1+yStg2)
yCtl=rnorm(N, mean=uCtl, sd=sy)
```

```
tValue=t.test(yTrt,yCtl)$statistic
if (tValue>=Zalpha) {power=power+1/nSims}
} ## End of i ##
return (c(power, probWinners))
}
```

Invoke the function:

```
## Determine critical value Zalpha for alpha (power) =0.025 ##
u0y=c(0,0,0); u0x=c(0,0,0)
powerBInfo(uCtl=0, u0y, u0x, rhou=1, suy=0, sux=0 ,rho=1, sy=4, sx=4,
Zalpha=2.772, N1=100, N=300, nArms=3, nSims=100000)
## Power simulation ##
u0y=c(1,0.5,0.2)
u0x=c(2,1,0.5)
powerBInfo(uCtl=0, u0y, u0x, rhou=0.2, suy=0.2, sux=0.2 ,rho=0.2, sy=4,
sx=4, Zalpha=2.772, N1=100, N=300, nArms=3, nSims=5000)
```

B.9   Chapter 10

```
##Chapter 10-Randomized Play-the-Winner Design with Binary Endpoint
## Randomized Play-the-Winner Design with Binary Endpoint
## a0, b0 = the initial numbers of balls for the two treatments A and B
## a1, b1 = balls added to the urn if a response is observed in arm A or arm
B
## RR1, RR2 = the response rates in groups 1 and 2
## nSbjs = total number of subjects (two groups combined)
## nMin (>0) = the minimum sample-size per group
## nAnlys = number of analyses
## interim analyses are designed for randomization adjustment
## aveP1 and aveP2 = the average response rates in groups 1 and 2
## Power = probability of the test statistic > Zc
RPWBinary = function(nSims=1000, Zc=1.96, nSbjs=200, nAnlys=3,
RR1=0.2, RR2=0.3, a0=1, b0=1, a1=1, b1=1, nMin=1) {
set.seed(21823)
Power=0; aveP1=0; aveP2=0; aveN1=0; aveN2=0
for (isim in 1:nSims) {
nResp1=0; nResp2=0; N1=0; N2=0
nMax=nSbjs-nMin
a=a0; b=b0; r0=a/(a+b)
for (iSbj in 1:nSbjs) {
```

```
nIA=round(nSbjs/nAnlys)
if (iSbj/nIA==round(iSbj/nIA)) {r0=a/(a+b)}
if ((rbinom(1,1,r0)==1 & N1<nMax) | N2>=nMax) {
N1=N1+1
if (rbinom(1,1,RR1)==1) {nResp1=nResp1+1; a=a+a1}
}
else
{
N2=N2+1
if (rbinom(1,1,RR2)==1) { nResp2=nResp2+1; b=b+b1 }
}
}
aveN1=aveN1+N1/nSims; aveN2=aveN2+N2/nSims
p1=nResp1/N1; p2=nResp2/N2
aveP1=aveP1+p1/nSims; aveP2=aveP2+p2/nSims
stdErr2=p1*(1-p1)/N1+p2*(1-p2)/N2
TS = (p2-p1)/sqrt(stdErr2)
if (TS>Zc) {Power=Power+1/nSims}
}
return (cbind(nSbjs, aveN1, aveN2, aveP1, aveP2, Zc, Power))
}
```

```
    RPWBinary(nSims=10000, Zc=2.01, nSbjs=200, nAnlys=1, RR1=0.4,
RR2=0.4, a0=1, b0=1,a1=0, b1=0, nMin=1)
    RPWBinary(nSims=1000, Zc=2.01, nSbjs=200, nAnlys=1, RR1=0.3,
RR2=0.5, a0=1, b0=1,a1=0, b1=0, nMin=1)
```

```
    RPWBinary(nSims=10000, Zc=2.035, nSbjs=200, nAnlys=5, RR1=0.4,
RR2=0.4, a0=2, b0=2,a1=1, b1=1, nMin=1)
    RPWBinary(nSims=1000, Zc=2.035, nSbjs=200, nAnlys=5, RR1=0.3,
RR2=0.5, a0=2, b0=2,a1=1, b1=1, nMin=1)
```

```
    RPWBinary(nSims=10000, Zc=2.010, nSbjs=200, nAnlys=200, RR1=0.4,
RR2=0.4, a0=1, b0=1,a1=0, b1=0, nMin=1)
    RPWBinary(nSims=1000, Zc=2.010, nSbjs=200, nAnlys=200, RR1=0.3,
RR2=0.5, a0=1, b0=1,a1=0, b1=0, nMin=1)
```

Chapter 10-Randomized Play-the-Winner Design with Normal Endpoint

```
    RARNorm=function(nSims=1000, nPts=100, nArms=5, b=1, m=1, Crt-
Max=1.96){
    AveN=rep(0,nArms); rP=rep(0,nArms); AveU=rep(0,nArms); PowerMax=0
    for (isim in 1:nSims){
```

```
        uObs=rep(0,nArms);        cuObs=rep(0,nArms);        Ns=rep(0,nArms);
Crp=rep(0,nArms)
    for (iSubject in 1:nPts) {
    for (i in 1:nArms){rP[i]=a0[i]+b*uObs[i]**m}
    Suma=0; for (i in 1:nArms){Suma=Suma+rP[i]}
    for (i in 1:nArms){rP[i]=rP[i]/Suma}
    CrP=rep(0,nArms)
    for (iArm in 1:nArms){
    for (i in 1:iArm){CrP[iArm]=CrP[iArm]+rP[i]}
    }
    rn=runif(1,0,1); cArm=1
    for (iArm in 2:nArms){
    if (CrP[iArm-1]<rn & rn<CrP[iArm]){cArm=iArm}
    }
    Ns[cArm]= Ns[cArm]+1
    ## For normal response
    u=rnorm(1, us[cArm],s[cArm])
    cuObs[cArm]=cuObs[cArm]+u
    for (i in 1:nArms){uObs[i]=cuObs[i]/max(Ns[i],1)}
    } ## End of iSubject
    se2=0
    ## Assume sigma known for simplicity
    for (i in 1:nArms){se2=se2+s[i]**2/max(Ns[i],1)*2/nArms}
    uMax=uObs[1]
    for (i in 1:nArms){if (uObs[i]>=uMax){iMax=i} }
    TSmax=(uObs[iMax]-uObs[1])*(Ns[1]+Ns[iMax])/2/(nPts/nArms)/se2**0.5
    if (TSmax>CrtMax){PowerMax=PowerMax+1/nSims}
    for (i in 1:nArms) {
    AveU[i]=AveU[i]+uObs[i]/nSims
    AveN[i]=AveN[i]+Ns[i]/nSims
    }
    } # End of iSim

    return (c("nPts=", nPts, "Power=", PowerMax, "AveN=", AveN, "AveU=",
AveU))
    }
```

Invoke the function:

```
    a0=rep(1,5); us=rep(0.06,5); s=rep(.18,5)
    RARNorm(nSims=10000, nPts=375, nArms=5, b=1, m=1, CrtMax=2.01)
    a0=rep(1,5); us=c(0.06, 0.12, 0.13, 0.14, 0.15); s=rep(.18,5)
    RARNorm(nSims=10000, nPts=375, nArms=5, b=1, m=1, CrtMax=2.01)
```

B.10   Chapter 11

```
## Chapter 11-CRM
    ## Trial simulation trial using CRM.
    ## b = model parameter in (11.1)
    ## aMin and aMax = the upper and lower limits of parameter a.
    CRM = function(nSims=100, nPts=30, nLevels=10, b=100, aMin=0.1,
        aMax=0.3,   MTRate=0.3,   nIntPts=100,   ToxModel="Skeleton",   nPts-
ForStop=6)
    {
    g0 = c(1); PercentMTD= c(1)
    DLTs=0; AveMTD=0; VarMTD=0; AveTotalN=0
    dx=(aMax-aMin)/nIntPts
    for (k in 1:nIntPts) {g0[k]=g[k]}
    PercentMTD=rep(0,nLevels)
    for (iSim in 1:nSims) {
    for (k in 1:nIntPts) {g[k]=g0[k]}
    nPtsAt=rep(0,nLevels); nRsps=rep(0,nLevels)
    iLevel=1; PreLevel=1
    for (iPtient in 1:nPts) {
    TotalN=iPtient
    TotalN=iPtient
    iLevel=min(iLevel, PreLevel+1); #Avoid dose-jump
    iLevel=min(iLevel, nLevels)
    PreLevel=iLevel;
    Rate=RRo[iLevel]
    nPtsAt[iLevel]=nPtsAt[iLevel]+1
    r= rbinom(1, 1, Rate)
    nRsps[iLevel]=nRsps[iLevel]+r
    # Posterior distribution of a
    c=0
    for (k in 1:nIntPts) {
    ak=aMin+k*dx
    if (ToxModel=="Logist") { Rate=1/(1+b*exp(-ak*doses[iLevel]))}
    if (ToxModel=="Skeleton") { Rate=skeletonP[iLevel]^exp(ak)}
    if (r>0) {L=Rate}
    if (r <= 0) {L=1-Rate}
    g[k]=L*g[k]; c=c+g[k]*dx
    }
    for (k in 1:nIntPts) {g[k]=g[k]/c}
    # Predict response rate and current MTD
    MTD=iLevel; MinDR=1; RR=rep(0, nLevels)
```

```
for (i in 1:nLevels) {
for (k in 1:nIntPts) {
ak=aMin+k*dx
if (ToxModel=="Logist") { RR[i]= RR[i]+1/(1+b*exp(-ak*doses[i]))*g[k]*dx}
if (ToxModel=="Skeleton") { RR[i]= RR[i]+skeletonP[i]^exp(ak)*g[k]*dx}
}
DR=abs(MTRate-RR[i])
if (DR<MinDR){MinDR=DR; iLevel=i;MTD = i}
}
if (nPtsAt[iLevel] >= nPtsForStop) {
PercentMTD[iLevel] =PercentMTD[iLevel]+1/nSims
break()
}
}
for (i in 1:nLevels) {DLTs=DLTs+nRsps[i]/nSims}
AveMTD=AveMTD+MTD/nSims
VarMTD=VarMTD+MTD^2/nSims
AveTotalN=AveTotalN+TotalN/nSims
}
SdMTD=sqrt(VarMTD-AveMTD^2)
return (cbind(AveTotalN, nLevels, AveMTD, SdMTD, DLTs))
}

#Logistic Model
g= c(1); doses = c(1)
RRo = c(0.01,0.02,0.03,0.05,0.12,0.17,0.22,0.4)
for (k in 1:100) {g[k]=1}; # Flat prior
for (i in 1:8) {doses[i]=i}
CRM(nSims=500, nPts=30, nLevels=8, b=150, aMin=0, aMax=3,
MTRate=0.17, ToxModel="Logist", nPtsForStop=6)
#Skeleton Model
g = c(1); doses = c(1)
RRo = c(0.01,0.02,0.03,0.05,0.12,0.17,0.22,0.4)
skeletonP=c(0.01,0.02,0.04,0.08,0.16,0.32,0.4,0.5)
for (k in 1:100) {g[k]=1}; # Flat prior
CRM(nSims=500, nPts=20, nLevels=8, aMin=-0.1, aMax=2,
MTRate=0.17, ToxModel="Skeleton", nPtsForStop=6)
```

B.11   Chapter 12

```
## Chapter 12 - Conditional Power
    ## EP = endpoint, "normal" or "binary"
    ## Model = "MSP", "MPP", or "MINP"
    ## alpha2 = 2nd stage stopping boundary on p-scale
    ## nStg2 = sample size at 2nd stage
    ## ux, uy = observed responses in the two groups
    ## p1 = interim p-value
    ## w1 = weight in MINP only
    ConPower=function(EP="normal", Model="MINP", alpha2=0.0226, ux=0.2,
uy=0.4, sigma=1, nStg2=100, p1=0.8, w1=0.707)
    {
    u=(ux+uy)/2
    if (EP=="binary"){sigma=(u*(1-u))**0.5}
    w2=sqrt(1-w1*w1)
    eSize=(uy-ux)/sigma
    if (Model=="MSP"){BFun=qnorm(1-max(0.0000001,alpha2-p1))}
    if (Model=="MPP"){BFun=qnorm(1-alpha2/p1)}
    if (Model=="MINP"){BFun=(qnorm(1-alpha2)- w1*qnorm(1-p1))/w2}
    cPower=1-pnorm(BFun-eSize*sqrt(nStg2/2))
    return (cPower)
    }
```

Invoke the function:

```
    ConPower(EP="binary", Model="MSP", alpha2=0.2050, ux=0.2, uy=0.4,
nStg2=100, p1=0.1)
    ConPower(EP="binary", Model="MPP", alpha2=0.0043, ux=0.2, uy=0.4,
nStg2=100, p1=0.1)
    ConPower(EP="binary", Model="MINP", alpha2=0.0226, ux=0.2, uy=0.4,
nStg2=100, p1=0.1, w1=0.707)
    ConPower(EP="normal", Model="MSP", alpha2=0.2050, ux=0.2, uy=0.4,
sigma=1, nStg2=200, p1=0.1)
    ConPower(EP="normal", Model="MPP", alpha2=0.0043, ux=0.2, uy=0.4,
sigma=1, nStg2=200, p1=0.1)
    ConPower(EP="normal", Model="MINP", alpha2=0.0226, ux=0.2, uy=0.4,
sigma=1, nStg2=200, p1=0.1, w1=0.707)
```

```
    ## Chapter 12 - New sample size at stage 2
    ## New sample size for stage 2
    ## trtDiff = observed treatment difference
    ## sigma = observed standard deviation
```

```
## p1 = p-value at the interim analysis
## NId = noninferiority margin
## cPower = targeted conditional power
## nStg2, n2New = initial and the new sample sizes for stage 2
NewN2byConditionalPowerForTwoStageSSR=function(trtDiff=0.5, sigma=1,
NId, p1, alpha2, nStg2, cPower, method="MINP", w1)
{
w2=sqrt(1-w1*w1)
if (method=="MSP") {BFun = qnorm(1-max(0.000001,alpha2-p1))}
if (method=="MPP") {BFun = qnorm(1- min(0.999999,alpha2/p1))}
if (method=="MINP"){BFun = (qnorm(1-alpha2)- w1*qnorm(1-p1))/w2}
eSize=(trtDiff+NId)/sigma
n2New=max(2*((BFun-qnorm(1-cPower))/eSize)^2, nStg2)
return (c("New sample at stage 2=", round(n2New)))
}
NewN2byConditionalPowerForTwoStageSSR(trtDiff=0.2, sigma=1.2, NId=0,
p1=0.1, alpha2=0.0226, nStg2=50, cPower=0.9, method="MINP", w1=0.707)
```

B.12 Chapter 13

```
## Chapter 13 - CRM Monitoring
## Trial monitoring using CRM.
## b = model parameter in (11.1)
## aMin and aMax = the upper and lower limits of parameter a
CRM = function(nSims=100, nPts=30, nLevels=10, b=100, aMin=0.1,
aMax=0.3, MTRate=0.3, nIntPts=100, ToxModel="Skeleton", nPts-
ForStop=6)
{
g0 = c(1); dx=(aMax-aMin)/nIntPts
for (k in 1:nIntPts) {g0[k]=g[k]}
## for (iSim in 1:nSims) {
for (k in 1:nIntPts) {g[k]=g0[k]}
nPtsAt=rep(0, nLevels); nRsps=rep(0, nLevels);
iLevel=1; PreLevel=1
for (iPtient in 1:nPts) {
TotalN=iPtient
TotalN=iPtient
iLevel=min(iLevel, PreLevel+1); #Avoid dose-jump
iLevel=min(iLevel, nLevels)
PreLevel=iLevel
Rate=RRo[iLevel]
```

```
nPtsAt[iLevel]=nPtsAt[iLevel]+1
## r= rbinom(1, 1, Rate) ## random Response
r=ObsResponses[iPtient] ## Observed response
nRsps[iLevel]=nRsps[iLevel]+r
## Posterior distribution of a
c=0
for (k in 1:nIntPts) {
ak=aMin+k*dx
if (ToxModel=="Logist") { Rate=1/(1+b*exp(-ak*doses[iLevel]))}
if (ToxModel=="Skeleton") { Rate=skeletonP[iLevel]^exp(ak)}
if (r>0) {L=Rate}
if (r <= 0) {L=1-Rate}
g[k]=L*g[k]; c=c+g[k]*dx
}
for (k in 1:nIntPts) {g[k]=g[k]/c}
# Predict response rate and current MTD
MTD=iLevel; MinDR=1
RR = rep(0,nLevels)
for (i in 1:nLevels) {
for (k in 1:nIntPts) {
ak=aMin+k*dx
if (ToxModel=="Logist") { RR[i]= RR[i]+1/(1+b*exp(-ak*doses[i]))*g[k]*dx}
if (ToxModel=="Skeleton") { RR[i]= RR[i]+skeletonP[i]^exp(ak)*g[k]*dx}
}
DR=abs(MTRate-RR[i])
if (DR<MinDR){MinDR=DR; iLevel=i;MTD = i}
}
if (nPtsAt[iLevel] >= nPtsForStop) {
break()
}
}

## } ## End of iSim
return (c("Dose Level=", PreLevel, "Predicted MTD=", MTD))
}
```

Invoke the function:

```
#Logistic Model
g= c(1); doses = c(1)
RRo = c(0.01,0.02,0.03,0.05,0.12,0.17,0.22,0.4)
ObsResponses=c(0,0,0,0,0,1,0,0,1,0,0)
for (k in 1:100) {g[k]=1}; # Flat prior
```

```
for (i in 1:8) {doses[i]=i}
CRM(nSims=500, nPts=11, nLevels=8, b=150, aMin=0, aMax=3,
MTRate=0.17, ToxModel="Logist", nPtsForStop=6)
#Skeleton Model
g = c(1); doses = c(1)
RRo = c(0.01,0.02,0.03,0.05,0.12,0.17,0.22,0.4)
skeletonP=c(0.01,0.02,0.04,0.08,0.16,0.32,0.4,0.5)
ObsResponses=c(0,0,0,0,0,1,0,0,1,0,0)
for (k in 1:100) {g[k]=1}; # Flat prior
CRM(nSims=500, nPts=11, nLevels=8, aMin=-0.1, aMax=2,
MTRate=0.17, ToxModel="Skeleton", nPtsForStop=6)
```

B.13   Chapter 14

```
## Chapter 14-GSD p-Value by Simulation
    ## GSD p-value by simulation based stagewise ordering
    ## u0, u1 = means for two treatment groups
    ## sigma0, sigma1 = standard deviations for two treatment groups
    ## n0Stg1, n1Stg1, n0Stg2, n1Stg2 = sample sizes for the two groups at stages
1 and 2
    ## alpha1 = efficacy stopping boundary at stage 1
    ## w1squared = weight squared for MINP only at stage 1
    ## nSims = the number of simulation runs
    ##pValue, pValue2 = p-value and conditional p-value at stage 2
Pvalue TwoStageGSDwithNormalEndpoint=function(u0,u1,sigma0,sigma1, n0Stg1,
n1Stg1, n0Stg2, n1Stg2, alpha1, w1squared=0.5, t2Obs=1.96, nSims=1000000)
    {
    pValue2=0; M=0; w1=sqrt(w1squared);
    for (i in 1:nSims) {
    y0Stg1=rnorm(1, u0, sigma0/sqrt(n0Stg1))
    y1Stg1=rnorm(1, u1, sigma1/sqrt(n1Stg1))
    z1=(y1Stg1-y0Stg1)/sqrt(sigma1**2/n1Stg1+sigma0**2/n0Stg1)
    t1=1-pnorm(z1)
    if(t1>alpha1) {
    M=M+1
    y0Stg2=rnorm(1, u0, sigma0/sqrt(n0Stg2))
    y1Stg2=rnorm(1, u1, sigma1/sqrt(n1Stg2))
    z2=(y1Stg2-y0Stg2)/sqrt(sigma1**2/n1Stg2+sigma0**2/n0Stg2)
    t2=w1*z1+sqrt(1-w1*w1)*z2
    if(t2>=t2Obs) {pValue2=pValue2+1}
```

```
}
}
pValue=alpha1+pValue2/nSims
pValue2=pValue2/M
return (c("pValue=", pValue, "pValue2=", pValue2))
}
```

Invoke the function:
Example 14.1
  PvalueTwoStageGSDwithNormalEndpoint(u0=0.05,u1=0.05,   sigma0=0.22, sigma1=0.22, n0Stg1=120, n1Stg1=120, n0Stg2=120, n1Stg2=120, alpha1=0.01, t2Obs=1.96)

B.14   Commonly Used Stopping Boundaries

For K-stage O'Brien-Fleming stopping boundaries with equal information for the interim analyses are summarized in Table C.1.

O'Brien-Fleming stopping boundaries for two-stage design using different information times are presented in Table C.2:

Table C.1: O'Brien-Fleming Stopping Boundaries on z-Scale with MINP

No. of Stages	α_1	α_2	α_3	α_4	α_5	α_6
2	2.7956	1.9768	—	—	—	—
3	3.4716	2.4548	2.0044	—	—	—
4	4.0485	2.8627	2.3374	2.0243	—	—
5	4.5606	3.2248	2.6331	2.2803	2.0396	—
6	5.0297	3.5565	2.9039	2.5148	2.2493	2.0533

Note: Obtained from ExpDesign Studio 5.0 $\alpha = 0.025$.

Table C.2: Two-Stage O'Brien-Fleming Stopping Boundaries with MINP

Info Time	1/5	1/4	1/3	2/5	1/2	2/3	3/4
α_1	2.8173	2.8129	2.8086	2.8043	2.7956	2.7848	2.7783
α_2	1.9921	1.9890	1.9860	1.9829	1.9768	1.9691	1.9645

Note: Obtained from ExpDesign Studio 5.0 $\alpha = 0.025$.

Bibliography

Armitage, P. (1955). Tests for linear trends in proportions and frequencies. *Biometrics*, 11:375–86.

Bauer, P. and Kohne K. (1994). Evaluation of experiments with adaptive interim analyses. *Biometrics*, 50:1029–1041.

Beck, R.W., Maguire, M.G., Bressler, N.M., Glassman, A.R., Lindblad A.S., and Ferris, F.L. (2007). Visual acuity as an outcome measure in clinical trials of retinal diseases. *Ophthalmology*, 2007 Oct; 114(10):1804–9.

Berry, D.A. et al. (2001). Adaptive Bayesian designs for dose-ranging drug trials. In *Case Studies in Bayesian Statistics V*, Gatsonis C., et al. (eds.). Springer-Verlag: New York, 99–181.

Biomarkers Definition Working Group (2001). Biomarkers and surrogate: preferred definitions and conceptual framework. *Clin Pharmacol Therapeutics*, 69:89–95.

Breslow, N.E. and Haug, C. (1977). Sequential comparison of exponential survival curves. *JASA*, 67:691–697.

Bretz, F. and Hothorn, L.A. (2002). Detecting dose-response using contrasts: asymptotic power and sample-size determination for binary data. *Statistics in Medicine*, 21:3325–3335.

Bretz, F., Pinheiro, J.C., and Branson, M. (2005). Combining multiple comparisons and modeling techniques in dose-response studies. *Biometrics*, 61:738–748.

Bretz, F. et al. (2006). Confirmatory seamless phase II/III clinical trials with hypotheses selection at interim: General concepts. *Biometrical Journal*, 48:4, 623–634 DOI: 10.1002 /bimj.200510232.

Brittain, E. and Hu, Z (2009). Noninferiority trial design and analysis with an ordered three-level categorical endpoint. *Journal of Biopharmaceutical Statistics*, 19:685–699.

Campbell, M.J., Julious, S.A. and Altman, D.G. (1995). Estimating sample sizes for binary, ordered categorical, and continuous outcomes in two group comparisons. *British Medical Journal*, 311:145–8.

Canner, P.L. (1997) Monitoring treatment differences in long-term clinical trials. *Biometrics*, 33:603–615.

Chakravarty, A. (2005). Regulatory aspects in using surrogate markers in clinical trials. In *The evaluation of surrogate endpoint*, Burzykowski, Molenberghs, and Buyse (eds.). Springer.

Chang, M. (2006a). Adaptive design based on sum of stagewise *p*-values. *Statistics in Medicine* (in press). DOI: 10.1002/sim.2755.

Chang, M. (2007a). Multiple-arm superiority and noninferiority designs with various endpoints. *Pharmaceutical Statistics*, 6:43–52. (www.interscience.wiley.com) DOI: 10.1002/pst.242

Chang, M. (2006b). Recursive two-stage adaptive design, submitted.

Chang, M., Chow, S.C., and Pong, A. (2006). Adaptive design in clinical research—Issues, opportunities, and recommendations. *Journal of Biopharm. Statistics*, 16:299–309.

Chang, M. (2007b). Multiple-endpoint adaptive design, submitted.

Chang, M. and Chow, S.C. (2005). A hybrid Bayesian adaptive design for dose response trials. *Journal of Biopharmaceutical Statistics*, 15:667–691.

Chang, M. and Chow, S.C. (2006). Power and sample-size for dose response studies. In *Dose Finding in Drug Development*, Ting, N. (ed.). Springer, New York.

Chang, M., Chow, S.C., and Pong, A. (2006). Adaptive design in clinical research – issues, opportunities, and recommendations. *Journal of Biopharmaceutical Statistics*, 16(3): 299–309.

Chang, M. (2007c). Adaptive Design Theory and Implementation Using SAS and R (Chapman & Hall/CRC Biostatistics Series). Chapman & Hall/CRC, Boca Raton, FL.

Chang, M. (2010). *Monte Carlo Simulation for the Pharmaceutical Industry*. Chapman & Hall/CRC: Boca Raton, FL.

Chang, M. (2011). *Modern Issues and Methods in Biostatistics*. Springer: New York.

Chang, M. and Wang, J. (2014). The add-arm design for unimodal response curve with unknown mode. *Journal of Biopharmaceutical Statistics*.

Chang, M. (2014). *Adaptive Design Theory and Implementation Using SAS and R*. 2nd Ed. Chapman & Hall/CRC: Boca Raton, FL.

Cheng, Y.S., Menon, S., and Chang, M. (2014). Group sequential design and monitoring using multivariate B-value tool for clinical trials with multiple co-primary endpoints. *Statistics in Biopharmaceutical Research*.

Cheng, Y. et al. (2014). Some recent advances in multivariate statistics: Modality inference and statistical monitoring of clinical trials with multiple co-primary endpoints. PhD Thesis, Boston University, graduate school of arts and sciences.

Cheng, Y. et al. (2014). Statistical Monitoring of Clinical Trials with Multiple Co-Primary Endpoints Using Multivariate B-value. 6(3):241–250.

Chevret, S. (Ed., 2006). Statistical methods for dose-finding experiments. John Wiley & Sons Ltd. West Sussex, England.

CHMP (2005). Guideline on the choice of the noninferiority margin, EMEA/EWP/2158/99. London, July 27, 2005.

CHMP (2009). Guideline on missing data in confirmatory clinical trials/1776/99 Rev. 1.

Chow, S.C. (2013). *Biosimilars: Design and Analysis of Follow-on Biologics*. Chapman and Hall/CRC: Boca Raton, FL.

Chow, S.C., Chang M., and Pong A. (2005). Statistical consideration of adaptive methods in clinical development. *Journal of Biopharmaceutical Statistics*, 15:575–91

Chow, S.C., Shao, J., and Wang, H. (2003). *Sample Size Calculation in Clinical Research*. Marcel Dekker, Inc., New York.

Chow, S.C., Shao, J., and Wang, H. (2011). *Sample Size Calculations in Clinical Research*, Second Edition. Chapman & Hall/CRC: Boca Raton, FL.

Chuang-Stein C. (2006). Sample size and the probability of a successful trial. *Pharmaceutical Statistics*, 5(4):305–309.

Chuang, S.C. and Agresti, A. (1997). A review of tests for detecting a monotone dose-response relationship with ordinal response data. *Statistics in Medicine*, 16: 2599–618.

Chuang, S.C. et al. (2006). Sample size re-estimation. *Drug Information Journal.*

Chuang-Stein, C., Stryszak, P., Dmitrienko, A., and W. Offen. (2007). Challenge of multiple co-primary endpoints: a new approach. *Statistics in Medicine*, 26(6):1181–1192.

Chuang-Stein, C. et al. (2013). Design and sample size consideration for global trials, In *Design and Analysis of Bridging Studies*, Liu, Chow, and Hsuao, (eds.). CRC: Boca Raton, FL.

Coad, D.S. and Rosenberger, W.F. (1999). A comparison of the randomized play-the-winner and the triangular test for clinical trials with binary responses. *Statistics in Medicine*, 18:761–769.

Cochran, W.G. (1954). Some methods for strengthening the common χ^2 tests. *Biometrics*, 10:417–51.

Conley, B.A. and Taube, S.E. (2004). Prognostic and predictive marker in cancer. *Disease Markers*. 20:35–43.

Cui, L., Hung, H.M.J., and Wang, S.J. (1999). Modification of sample-size in group sequential trials. *Biometrics*, 55:853–857.

De Gruttola, V.G. et al. (2001). Considerations in the evaluation of surrogate endpoints in clinical trials: Summary of a National Institutes of Health Workshop. controlled clinical trials. 22:485–502.

Dowlman, N. (2001). Intelligent Medication Management-Using IVR to Optimise the Drug Supply Process. *Pharmaceutical Manufacturing and Packaging Sourcer*, (Summer) 24–28.

Dragalin V. (2006). Adaptive Designs: Terminology and Classification. *Drug Information Journal*, 40(4):425–436. 13.

Dragalin, V. and Fedorov, V. (2006). Adaptive designs for dose-finding based on efficacy–toxicity response. *Journal of Statistical Planning and Inference*, 136:1800–1823.

Dragalin, V., Fedorov, V., and Wu, Y. (2008). Adaptive designs for selecting drug combinations based on efficacy-toxicity response. *Journal of Statistical Planning and Inference*, 138:352–373.

Dunnett, C.W. (1955). A multiple comparison procedure for comparing several treatments with a control. *Journal of the American Statistical Association*, 50:1096–121.

Dunnett C.W. (1964). New tables for multiple comparisons with a control. *Biometrics*, 20:482–491.

Ellenberg, S.S., Fleming, T.R., and DeMets, D.L. (2002). Data Monitoring Committees in Clinical Trials – A Practical Perspective, John Wiley and Sons, New York, New York.

European Medicines Agency (EMEA). (2002). Point to Consider on Methodological Issues in Confirmatory Clinical Trials with Flexible Design and Analysis Plan. The European Agency for the Evaluation of Medicinal Products Evaluation of Medicines for Human Use. CPMP/EWP/2459/02, London, UK.

EMEA (2004). Point to Consider on the Choice of Non-inferiority Margin. The European Agency for the Evaluation of Medicinal Products Evaluation of Medicines for Human Use. London, UK.

EMEA (2005). Committee for Medicinal Products for Human Use (CHMP). Guideline on the Evaluation of Anticancer Medicinal Products in Man. December 2005. Available from http:// www.emea.eu.int /pdfs/human/ewp/ 020595en.pdf. Date of access: 10 August 2006.

EMEA (2006). Reflection Paper on Methodological Issues in Confirmatory Clinical Trials with Flexible Design and Analysis Plan. The European Agency for the Evaluation of Medicinal Products Evaluation of Medicines for Human Use. CPMP/EWP/2459/02, London, UK.

Emerson, S.S. (1988). Parameter estimation following group sequential hypothesis testing. PhD dissertation. University of Washington.

Emerson, S.S. and Fleming, T.R. (1990). Parameter estimation following group sequential hypothesis testing. *Biometrika*, 77:875–892.

Emerson, S.S. and Kittelson, J.M. (1997). A computationally simpler algorithm for the UMVUE of a normal mean following a group sequential test. *Biometrics*, 53:365–369.

Fairbanks, K. and Madsen, R. (1982). p-Values for tests using a repeated significance test design. *Biometrika*, 69:69–74.

FDA (1988). Guideline for Format and Content of the Clinical and Statistical Sections of New Drug Applications. The United States Food and Drug Administration, Rockville, Maryland.

FDA (2000). Guidance for Clinical Trial Sponsors on the Establishment and Operation of Clinical Trial Data Monitoring Committees. The United States Food and Drug Administration, Rockville, Maryland.

FDA (2005). Guidance for Clinical Trial Sponsors. Establishment and Operation of Clinical Trial Data Monitoring Committees (Draft). Rockville, Maryland. http://www.fda.gov/ cber/qdlns/ clintrialdmc.htm.

FDA (March 2006). Innovation Stagnation, Critical Path Opportunities List. www.fda.gov

FDA Guidance for Industry (draft). Clinical Trial Endpoints for the Approval of Cancer Drug and Biologiecs. FDA, April, 2005. Available from URL: http://www.fda.gov/cder/Guidance/6592dft.htm. Date of access: 11 August 2006.

FDA. Draft Guidance for the Use of Bayesian Statistics in Medical Device Clinical Trials. www.fda.gov/cdrh/osb/guidance/1601.pdf. Accessed 22 May 2006.

FDA. Providing Clinical Evidence of Effectiveness for Human Drug and Biological Products, Guidance for Industry [online]. Available from URL: http://www.fda.gov/cder/guidance/index.htm [Accessed 2005 July 20]

FDA (2010). Guidance for Industry Non-Inferiority Clinical Trials (draft). Food and Drug Administration, Department of Health and Human Services: Washington, DC.

Fisher, M.R., Roecker, E.B., and DeMets, D.L. (2001). The role of an independent statistical analysis center in the industry-modified national institutes of health model. *Drug Information Journal*, 35:115–129.

Friede, T. and Kieser, M. (2003). Blinded sample size reassessment in non-inferiority and equivalence trials. *Statistics in Medicine*, 22:995–1007.

Friede, T. and Kieser, M. (2006). Sample size recalculation in internal pilot study designs: A review. *Biometrical Journal*, 48:537–555.

Friede, T., Parsons, N., Stallard, N., Todd, S., Valdes, M.E., Chataway, J., and Nicholas, R. (2011). Designing a seamless phase II/III clinical trial using early outcomes for treatment selection: An application in multiple sclerosis. *Statistics in Medicine*, 30(13):1528–40.

Gallo, P. (2006). Operational challenges in adaptive design implementation. *Pharmaceutical Statistics*, 5:119–24.

Gaydos, B. et al. (2006). Adaptive dose response studies. *Drug Information Journal*, 40(4):451–461.

Gould, A.L. (1992). Interim analyses for monitoring clinical trials that do not maternally affect the type-I error rate. *Statistics in Medicine*, 11:55–66.

Gould, A.L. (1995). Planning and revising the sample-size for a trial. *Statistics in Medicine*, 14:1039–1051.

Gould, A.L. and Shih, W.J. (1992). Sample size re-estimation without unblinding for normally distributed outcomes with unknown variance. *Communications in Statistics - Theory and Methods*, 21:2833–2853.

Gould, A.L. and Shih, W.J. (1998). Modifying the design of ongoing trials without unblinding. *Statistics in Medicine*, 17:89–100.

Hamilton, S. and Ho, K.F. (2004). Efficient drug supply algorithms for stratified clinical trials by focusing on patient coverage–not just site supplies–this dynamic approach significantly reduces drug waste. *Applied Clinical Trials*, Feb 1, 2004.

Huang, W.S., Liu, J.P, and Hsiao, C.F. (2011). An alternative phase II/III design for continuous endpoints. *Pharmaceutical Statistics*, 10:105–114

Ivanova, A. and Flournoy, N. (2001). A birth and death urn for ternary outcomes: stochastic processes applied to urn models. In *Probability and Statistical Models with Applications*, Charalambides, C.A., Koutras, M.V., and Balakrishnan, N. (eds.). Chapman and Hall/CRC Press, Boca Raton, Florida, 583–600.

Ivanova, A., Liu, K., Snyder, E., and Snavely, D. (2009). An adaptive design for identifying the dose with the best efficacy/tolerability profile with application to a crossover dose finding study. *Statistics in Medicine*, 28:2941–2951.

Ivanova, A. and Wang, K. (2004). A non-parametric approach to the design and analysis of two-dimensional dose-finding trials. *Statistics in Medicine*, 23(12):1861–1870.

Ivanova, A., Xiao, C., and Tymofyeyev, Y. (2012). Two-stage designs for phase 2 dose-finding trials. *Statistics in Medicine*, 31:2872–2881.

Jenkins, M., Stone, A., and Jennison, C. (2010). An adaptive seamless phase II/III design for oncology trials with subpopulation selection using correlated survival endpoints. *Pharmaceutical Statistics*, 10:347–356.

Jennison, C. and Turnbull, B.W. (2000). *Group Sequential Tests with Applications to Clinical Trials*, Chapman & Hall: London/Boca Raton, Florida.

Jones, B. and Kenward, M. (2003). *Design and Analysis of Cross-Over Trials*, Second Edition. Chapman & Hall/CRC: Boca Raton, FL.

Julious, S.A. (2004). Tutorial in biostatistics:Sample sizes for clinical trials with normal data. *Statistics in Medicine*, 23:1921–86.

Lachin, J.M. and Foukes, M.A. (1986). Evaluation of sample-size and power for analysis of survival with allowance for nonuniform patient entry, losses to follow-up, noncompliance, and stratification. *Biometrics*, 42:507–19.

Lee, B.L and Fan, S.K. (2012). A two-dimensional search algorithm for dose-finding trials of two agents. *Journal of Biopharmaceutical Statistics*, 22(4):802–18.

Lehmacher, W. and Wassmer G. (1999). Adaptive sample-size calculations in group sequential trials. *Biometrics*, 55:1286–1290.

Li, W.J., Shih, W.J. and Wang, Y. (2005), Two-stage adaptive design for clinical trials with survival data. *Journal of Biopharmaceutical Statistics*, 15:707–718.

Li, G., Zhu, J., Ouyang, S.P., Xie, J., Deng, L., Law, G. (2009). Adaptive designs for interim dose selection. *Statistics in Biopharmaceutical Research*, 1(4):366–76.

Lin, Y. and Shih, W. J. (2001). Statistical properties of the traditional algorithm-based designs for phase I cancer clinical trials. *Biostatistics*, 2:203–215.

Little, R.J. (2010). *Panel on Handling Missing Data in Clinical Trial: The Prevention and Treatment of Missing Data in Clinical Trials.* The National Academies Press: Washington, D.C.

Little, R.J. and Rubin, D.B. (2002). *Statistical Analysis with Missing Data*, 2nd edition. Wiley: New York.

Liu, Q. and Chang, M. (2010). Note on Special Technical Issue on Adaptive Designs for Clinical Trials. In Special Issue: Adaptive Designs for Clinical Trials: Considerations about and Beyond the FDA Adaptive Designs Guidance.

Looker A.C., Dallman P.R., Carroll M.D., Gunter E.W., Johnson C.L. (1997). Prevalence of iron deficiency in the United States. JAMA 277:973–976

Maca, J. et al. (2006). Adaptive seamless phase II/III designs – background, operational aspects, and examples. *Drug Information Journal*, 40:463–473, 2006 • 0092-8615/2006.

Machin, D. et al. (1997). Statistical tables for the design of clinical studies. Ed. 2. Blackwell Scientific Publications: Oxford.

McEntegart, D. (2003). Forced Randomization When Using Interactive Voice Response Systems. *Applied Clinical Trials*, October 2003, 50–58.

Meyerson, L., Muirhead, R., Stryszak, P. et al. (2007). Multiple co-primary endpoints: Medical and statistical solutions a report from the multiple endpoints expert team of the pharmaceutical research and manufacturers of america. *Drug information journal*, 41:31–46.

Miller, F., Guilbaud, O., and Dette, H. (2007). Optimal designs for estimating the interesting part of a dose-effect curve. *Journal of Biopharmaceutical Statistics*, 17:1097–1115.

Nadarajah, S. and Kotz, S. (2008). Exact distribution of the max/min of two Gaussian random variables. *IEEE Transactions on Very Large Sclae Integration (VLSI) System*, vol. 16, no. 2.

Nam, J (1997). Establishing equivalence of two treatments and sample size requirements in matched-pairs design. *Biometrics*, 53:1422–1430.

O'Quigley, J., Pepe, M., and Fisher, L. (1990). Continual reassessment method: A practical design for phase I clinical trial in cancer. *Biometrics*, 46:33–48.

O'Quigley, J. and Shen, L. (1996). Continual reassessment method: A likelihood approach. *Biometrics*, 52:673–684.

Pocock, S.J. (2005). When (not) to stop a clinical trial for benefit. *Journal of American Medical Association*, 294:2228–2230.

Posch, M., Maurer, W., and Bretz, F. (2011). Type I error rate control in adaptive designs for confirmatory clinical trials with treatment selection at interim. *Pharmaceutical Statistics*, 10:96–104.

Proschan, M.A. (2005). Two-stage sample-size re-estimation based on a nuisance parameter: a review. *Journal of Biopharmaceutical Statistics*, 15:559–574.

Quinlan, J.A., Gallo, P., and Krams, M. (2006). Implementing adaptive designs: logistical and operational consideration. *Drug Information*, 40(4): 437–444.

Rosner, G. L. and Tsiatis, A. A. (1988). Exact confidence intervals following a group sequential trial: A comparison of methods. *Biometrika*, 75:723–729.

Ruberg, S.J. (1998). Contrasts for identifying the minimum effective dose. *Journal of the American Statistical Association*, 84:816–22.

Shih, W.J. and Lin, Y.(2006). Traditional and modified algorithm-based designs for phase I cancer clinical trials. in Cheveret S. (Ed., 2006). Statistical methods for dose-finding experiments. John Wiley & Sons. New York, New York.

Shun, Z., Lan, G., and Soo, Y. (2008). Interim treatment selection using the normal approximation approach in clinical trials. *Statistics in Medicine*, 27:597—618

Stallard, N. (2010). A confirmatory seamless phase II/III clinical trial design incorporating short-term endpoint information. *Statistics in Medicine*, 29(9): 959–71.

Stewart, W. and Ruberg, S.J. (2000). Detecting dose response with contrasts. *Statistics in Medicine*, 19:913–21.

Tang, D. and Geller, N.L. (1999). Closed testing procedures for group sequential clinical trials with multiple endpoints. *Biomatrics*, 55:1188–1192.

Ting, N. (2006) (Ed.). Dose Finding in drug development. Springer Science+Business Media Inc., N.Y.

Todd, S. and Stallard, N. (2005). A new clinical trial design combining phases 2 and 3: sequential designs with treatment selection and a change of endpoint. *Drug Information Journal*, 39:109–118.

Torres, M. and Moayedi, S. (2007). Evaluation of the acutely dyspneic elderly patient. *Clinics in Geriatric Medicine*, 23 (2):307–25, vi.

Tsagris, M., Beneki, C., and Hassani, H. (2014). On the Folded Normal Distribution. *Mathematics*, 2(1):12–28.

Tsiatis, A.A. and Mehta, C. (2003). On the inefficiency of the adaptive design for monitoring clinical trials. *Biometrika*, 90:367–378.

Tsiatis, A.A., Rosner G.L., and Metha, C.R. (1984). Exact confidence intervals following a group sequential test. *Biometrics*, 40:797–803.

Tukey, J.W. and Heyse, J.F. (1985). Testing the statistical certainty of a response to increasing doses of a drug. *Biometrics*, 41:295–301.

Walton, M.K. (2006). PhRMA-FDA Adaptive Design Workshop.

Wang, J., Chang M., Menon S., and Wang L. (2013). Biomarker informed adaptive seamless phase II/III design. JBS, submitted.

Wang, S.J., Hung, H.M.J., and O'Neill, R.T. (2006). Adapting the sample-size planning of a phase III trial based on phase II data. *Pharmaceutical Statistics*, 5:85–97.

Wang, S.K. and Tsiatis, A.A. (1987). Approximately optimal one-parameter boundaries for a sequential trials. *Biometrics*, 43:193–200.

Wei, L.J. (1977). A class of designs for sequential clinical trials. *Journal of American Statistical Association*, 72:382–386.

Wei, L.J. (1978). The adaptive biased-coin design for sequential experiments. *Annals of Statistics*, 9:92–100.

Wei, L.J. and Durham, S. (1978). The randomized play-the-winner rule in medical trials. *Journal of American Statistical Association*, 73:840–843.

Williams, D.A. (1971). A test for difference between treatment means when several dose levels are compared with a zero dose control. *Biometrics*, 27:103–17.

Williams, D.A. (1972). Comparison of several dose levels with a zero dose control. *Biometrics*, 28:519–31.

Wittes, J. and Brittain, E. (1990). The role of internal pilot studies in increasing the efficiency of clinical trials. *Statistics in Medicine*, 9:65–72.

Wittes, J., Schabenberger, O., Zucker, D., Brittain, E., and Proschan, M. (1999). Internal pilot studies I: type I error rate of the naive t-test. *Statistics in Medicine*, 18:3481–3491.

Yin, G. and Yuan, S. (2011). Bayesain approach for adaptive design, in Handbook of Adaptive Designs in Pharmaceutical and Clinical Development, Edited by Pong, A. and Chow, S.C. CRC Press, Taylor & Francis Group. Boca Raton, FL.

Zucker, D.M. et al. (1999). Internal pilot studies II: comparison of various procedures. *Statistics in Medicine*, 19:901–911.

Index

Note: Page numbers ending in "f" refer to figures. Page numbers ending in "t" refer to tables.